Epidemiological Research

Mbuso Mabuza

Published by Mbuso Mabuza, 2022.

While every precaution has been taken in the preparation of this book, the publisher assumes no responsibility for errors or omissions, or for damages resulting from the use of the information contained herein.

EPIDEMIOLOGICAL RESEARCH

First edition. September 12, 2022.

Copyright © 2022 Mbuso Mabuza.

ISBN: 979-8201913205

Written by Mbuso Mabuza.

Also by Mbuso Mabuza

A Healthy Mind And Best You: Achieving Great Results in Every Aspect of Your Life

Purposeful And Better You

Sustainable Development Calls for Effective Strategic Leadership for Efficient Health Systems

Health Promotion In Low Socioeconomic Settings

Medicine and Sociology of Health

Qualitative Methods In Public Health Research

Epidemiological Research

Ethics, Qualitative And Quantitative Methods In Public Health Research

Table of Contents

Preface

This book provides an introduction to epidemiological research and statistical methods covering key concepts and all the main types of epidemiological study. It elicits a critical understanding of the purpose and context of quantitative research including the basis for selecting appropriate research designs from a thorough grounding in the uses and methods of epidemiology; key statistical concepts and techniques needed for the basic analysis of data; critical evaluation of statistical and epidemiological techniques in health research.

The book has been designed around a number of core published information dealing with various topics from the United Kingdom, Europe and the low- and middle-income countries. These studies have been chosen to introduce you to a wide range of study methods. The main intriguing aspects of their design provide examples which are used to help you understand the fundamental principles of good research, and to practise these techniques yourself.

The topics covered in this book include the following: scientific method and introductory concepts; routine data sources and descriptive epidemiology; surveys; cohort studies; case-control studies; and critical appraisal of research evidence.

This book will be a valuable resource to health professionals, researchers, statisticians, data scientists, health programmers, policymakers, medical students, graduate and postgraduate students in public health and related disciplines.

Dr Mbuso Mabuza

Global Health, Medicine and International Public Health Consultant

Chapter 1

Scientific Method and Introductory Concepts

This chapter will cover the following topics:

- Approaches to scientific research
- Epidemiology, incidence, prevalence, and the concepts of prevention

1.1 Approaches to scientific research

IT HAS ALWAYS MADE one wonder why certain schools of thought are more dominant and more acceptable than others when it comes to research approaches. Bruce, Pope & Stanistreet (2008) acknowledge that paradigm shifts, social influences and experiences have had a huge bearing on how research has been conducted over the years. Although the status quo indicates that the dominant fields of biomedicine and epidemiology follow a positivist approach while the less dominant social sciences follow an interpretative approach, there is an emerging discourse which promotes a combination of research approaches (Johnson, Onwuegbuzie & Turner, 2007). As such, one's research experiences/interests to date might influence the way in which one decides to design and carry out future research.

Suppose one's career started in the biomedical sciences, and the only research approach used was a positivist approach, whereby all our research projects were conducted by following quantitative research methods. For example, if one was involved with molecular research and also spent some time in the cancer research laboratory whereby a series of laboratory analyses on glutathione-dependent metabolism of certain anticancer drugs were conducted. In such cases, quantitative research methods were the most ideal because there was an obligation to measure and to make calculations based on the molecular systems that we were dealing with.

After having qualified as a bio-chemical scientist and physician, and having gained clinical and community experience, one realised that human beings are more complex and unique. Although one still saw the important role of biomedical science and 'mainstream' medicine, one also felt that this was not enough because there was still much more that we did not understand about the uniqueness and complexity of human beings and about what makes them healthy or unhealthy. Human beings respond differently to similar stressors, diseases, disasters, and treatment. Hence, the need to follow an interpretative research approach that could explore and tap into the uniqueness of human beings and about what makes them healthy or unhealthy, without having to follow a formalized and standardized quantitative approach. One has subsequently completed a few qualitative research studies at different firms and communities of southern Africa, in order to explore the perceptions of people about the effectiveness of organisational health and wellbeing, social and economic empowerment, health strategies and programmes, among others. Lesson learnt was that not everything about human beings can be measured or generalized, especially when it comes to issues of health. Da Costa & French (1990) report that formalized models are not everything when it comes to health research. Sachs & Kranz (1997) highlight the importance of anthropology and sociology when studying a medical problem.

Certainly, one research approach cannot provide all the answers. As such, both an epidemiological and a socio-economic research perspective will be of value not only to the local community, but to the country, the region and beyond, in terms of interventions. A paradigm shift is necessary if we are to make a significant contribution to health, but this will require the methodological wrangles between the positivist and interpretative proponents to be minimized, in order to create an enabling environment for harmonisation, innovation and positive impact for health (Popay & Williams, 1996).

It is a pity that purists often believe that their way is the best way or the only way, and that their paradigm cannot coexist with another. There is no doubt that the positivist paradigm in research has enjoyed great dominance over the years and this has entrenched the agenda of quantitative research methods with the belief that research must be limited to what can be observed and measured objectively (Joubert & Ehrlich,2007) . It has been highlighted that Thomas Kuhn (1922-1996) popularized the idea of a paradigm and mentioned that any dominant paradigm is bound to be challenged and replaced by another at some point in time (Bruce et al, 2008). It is hardly surprising that the positivist paradigm has been challenged by social scientists and other interpretative proponents who argue that human behaviour cannot be simply reduced to a mere value or statistic (Welman et al, 2005).

Human beings need to be understood not only from a positivist perspective, but from a holistic perspective, and a mixed research approach could be of benefit in that regard. Philosophers such as Charles Sanders Peirce and John Dewey advocate a pragmatic stance in research (Johnson & Onwuegbuzie 2004). The weaknesses of one paradigm could be complemented by the strengths of the other paradigm. For example, during one's time as a field researcher to determine the effectiveness of family planning methods in the rural, urban and industrial settings of the Kingdom of Eswatini, one realized that both approaches nicely complemented each other. In addition to making quantitative analyses, we were able to qualitatively gain an insight into why people behaved the way they did according to their own experiences in their own settings. This helped in understanding local factors such as human experiences and other factors, for intervention purposes (Sachs & Kranz, 1997).

Moreover, both research paradigms are important, and the unique strengths of each paradigm could benefit the overall human behaviour research discourse. It is interesting to observe that there are many researchers who have now realized the importance of having an integrated research approach. Johnson & Onwuegbuzie (2004) observe that contrary to purists' beliefs, the two paradigms have important similarities such as empirical observations and use of safeguards, which are an opportunity to strengthen the new discourse of a mixed method research approach.

It is imperative that proponents of the two research paradigms get their house in order for a common purpose as we are now faced with new situations in public health research and practice (Popay & Williams, 1996). We need to be open-minded and transcend the disciplinary boundaries and realize that there are other ways of conducting research, which could benefit the overall health research and thereby balance the communication and understanding of human behaviour research (Rosenfield, 1992). However, it has to be acknowledged that human behaviour cannot be completely understood as human beings are unique and influenced by complex factors.

It is a scary reality that the force of gravity is pulling us in one direction, as we have to make do with what we have at our disposal, and what we think is the best science of our time. The good thing is that science is not fixed as it is always evolving, and as it evolves we also evolve and hopefully gain a better understanding. At the same time, one wonders if what we consider as the best science of our time is indeed the best science of our time. Is there a possibility that most published health research findings will be proved wrong in the future as the paradigm of scientific research evolves? One will probably say yes, because one believes that nothing is absolute in this world.

There are many things that cannot be measured using the current scientific methods. In fact, there is a lot that we still do not understand about life. Some scholars acknowledge that epidemiology does not seek to find proof, but seeks to find associations, even though epidemiologists put more emphasis on empiricism. However, there are times when the epidemiologist takes things for granted and believes that everything must be evidence based (Bruce et al, 2008). Similarly, there are times when those who follow a qualitative scientific approach also take things for granted and conduct their research with a perceived agenda with regard to the research question instead of first getting to understand the needs of the target population (Maghboeba et al, 2005).

It gets fascinating at times to observe the power of the media in driving the agenda of evidence-based medicine or science which derives from the scientific notion that everything must be objectively measured and tested to prove its efficacy. The issue of evidence-base has had a huge bearing on research funding. Anything that is portrayed to be outside the scope of the evidence base is often side-lined. Money can affect the norms and the philosophy of science especially with the involvement of the multi-billion pharmaceutical industry in health care research and funding. Political lobbying can also influence the dimension and direction of the philosophy of science as this can influence the national or international health budget which can sway the power in favour of what is considered an acceptable scientific paradigm of that particular time.

When one reflects on the work of French philosophers such as Deleuze and Guattari, one realizes that health sciences are outrageously exclusionary and dangerously normative when it comes to scientific knowledge and scientific research (Holmes et al, 2006). It was interesting to read a few articles reporting that the majority of published research results are false, but they are accurate based on the prevailing scientific bias or paradigm (Ioannidis, 2005).

1.2 Epidemiology, Incidence, prevalence, and the concepts of prevention

THERE ARE MANY GOOD definitions of epidemiology that have been proposed. However, the one that captures the spirit in the context of public health research is: 'epidemiology is the study of the distribution and determinants of health-related states or events in specific populations, and the application of this study to the control of health problems' (Dictionary of epidemiology, 2001). As such, epidemiology is not about individuals, but it is a population science.

Statistics is a discipline which includes empirical and estimated quantitative data, and the classification of such data according to probability theory and hypothesis testing (World Health Organization, 2018). For example, health statistics includes empirical data and estimates related to health, such as mortality, morbidity, risk factors, among others, to display, summarise and compare data, and makes it possible to make inferences about a population or populations (World Health Organization, 2018). Experts in statistics sometimes regard statistics about births, mortality, marriages and divorces as vital statistics (U.S. National Library of Medicine, 2017).

Epidemiology and statistics are related in the sense that epidemiology is a quantitative discipline which relies on statistical approaches or models to analyse data, applicable to sound research methods.

Scenarios of incidence and prevalence

- The term incidence in relation to angina could be explained as the number of new cases of angina in a defined at risk population in a specified period of time; whereas, prevalence is all the cases of angina that existed in that defined at risk population at that particular point in time or during that specified period (Bruce et al, 2008).

- This might be because prevalence includes all the cases of angina that existed in 2009 including cases of angina that existed at the start of 2009 and new cases that occurred during 2009. Joubert & Ehrlich (2007) refer to this type of prevalence as period prevalence. On the other hand, the incidence of angina excludes cases of angina that existed at the start of 2009 and only included new cases of angina that occurred during the course of 2009. Unlike prevalence, incidence often focuses on a smaller population (Waraich et al, 2004). Nevertheless, both prevalence and incidence are useful ways of measuring disease frequency (Gavin et al, 2005).

- Calculation of the prevalence of psychiatric disorder in residential care:

Prevalence = Number of cases at a given time/Number in population at that time (Bruce et al, 2008)

Given number of cases at a given time = 198

Given number in population = 2,790

This implies that prevalence = 198/2,790 = 0.07

Therefore, the prevalence of psychiatric disorder amongst those in residential care is 7 per cent or 70 per 1000

- Calculation of the prevalence of psychiatric disorder in foster care:

Prevalence = Number of cases at a given time/Number in population at that time (Bruce et al, 2008)

Given number of cases at a given time = 324

Given number in population = 8,390

This implies that prevalence = 324/8,390 = 0.039

Therefore, the prevalence of psychiatric disorder amongst those in foster care is 3.9 per cent or 39 per 1000

Scenarios of the concepts of prevention

1.	Offering alendronate (a drug to prevent osteoporotic fragility fractures) to women with osteoporosis to prevent fracture	Tertiary prevention
2.	Screening using mammography to identify the presence of early breast cancer and subsequent treatment of positive cases	Secondary prevention
3.	Approaches such as smoking prevention and cessation treatments in a group of asymptomatic smokers to reduce the risk of lung cancer	Primary prevention
4.	In a group of patients suffering from incontinence, carrying out bladder training exercises to prevent the condition from worsening	Tertiary prevention
5.	The application of dental sealants in school children to prevent tooth decay	Primary prevention
6.	Faecal occult blood testing to screen for colon cancer to reduce the incidence and mortality of colon cancer through the detection and removal of precancerous polyps	Secondary prevention
7.	Early detection and treatment of diabetic eye disease to reduce the possibility of blindness in patients with diabetes	Tertiary prevention
8.	Palliative care in patients with bowel cancer to reduce inflammation (corticosteroids) and pain (morphine)	Tertiary prevention
9.	Establishing an antibacterial water treatment intervention to provide safe drinking water in a village in Guatemala and reduce the occurrence of diarrhoea in children in the village	Primary prevention
10.	Prescription of anti-inflammatory drugs in patients with rheumatoid arthritis to improve range of movement and reduce pain	Tertiary prevention

It is possible that the discovery and provision of antiretroviral drugs (ARVs) as treatment for HIV has been both a blessing and a curse.

The blessing has been significant as ARVs have kept people who are living with HIV, healthy, and reduced the chance of passing HIV on to others. As such, ARVs have given hope to individuals, families, communities, workplaces, nations, and the world at large, as huge reductions in transmission, morbidity and mortality rates have been seen where antiretroviral therapy (ART) has been used correctly and consistently.

The curse has manifested in a number of ways, particularly in the heavily disease-burdened southern Africa region, and other disease burdened regions in different parts of the world. Firstly, knowing that many people who take ARVs as treatment can live for many years, and that those who take ARVs as prevention (such as pre-exposure prophylaxis - PrEP, and/or post-exposure prophylaxis - PEP) could result in people reverting to risky sexual behaviour or risky drug injecting behaviour with the comfort that there are ARVs available. Such risky behaviour could become fertile ground for further spread of HIV. Secondly, the ARVs are very expensive, and most of the countries south of the Sahara are poor and cannot sustain the supply of ARVs, and as such, lack of sustainable supply could compound the challenge of poor adherence to treatment. Thirdly, a huge chunk of the health budget of most southern African countries is channelled towards HIV and AIDS, and this somewhat compromises other key strategic and programmatic areas that need urgent attention such as the epidemic of non-communicable diseases and emerging/or re-emerging infectious diseases (Sewankambo & Katamba, 2009).

In 2014, the news that the "Mississippi Baby" who was put on antiretroviral treatment within 30 hours of birth and was supposedly "cured" of HIV, was met with great excitement and celebration by the majority of people worldwide. Similarly, there was great excitement and belief that scientists were very close to finding a cure for HIV when it was reported at the 9th International IAS Conference on HIV Science, in Paris, 23-26 July 2017, that a nine-year old South African child with HIV at birth and who had been off antiretroviral drugs for eight and a half years showed no symptoms or signs of active HIV. To see such great joy in the faces of many people was really very interesting because it made one realize the magnitude and the impact those positive stories had made. If scientific research could come up with a cure for HIV, who will really benefit? Some studies report that it is the scientific innovators or the drug producers that would benefit the most because there will always be a huge demand particularly from the middle- and low-income countries where there is the heaviest burden of HIV and AIDS (Philipson & Jena, 2005).

When we talk about a cure, it makes one think, because we seem to live in a society which believes that everything must have a cure. The concern is that in due course, the cure is bound to fail or result in therapeutic drug resistance, which means, scientific research must again look for another cure to deal with an even tougher "monster" that has been created. For example, it is a known fact that mycobacterium tuberculosis (TB) can be cured. However, there are already tougher "monsters" such as multi-drug resistant tuberculosis (MDR-TB) and extreme drug resistant tuberculosis (XDR-TB) cases that we have already seen. Is a cure for HIV not going to create another tougher "monster"? Only time will tell. The bottom line is that prevention is better than cure. Primary prevention is the most preferred because it prevents a disease from the beginning, then secondary prevention, and lastly, tertiary prevention (Bruce et al, 2008).

References

Bruce, N., Pope, D. & Stanistreet, D. (2008) Philosophy of science and introduction to epidemiology'. In: *Quantitative research methods for health research: a practical guide to epidemiology*. Chichester: John Wiley & Sons, Ltd.

Da Costa, N.C.A. & French, S. (1990) 'The model-theoretic approach in the philosophy of Science', *Philosophy of Science*, 57 (2), pp. 248-265.

Gavin, N., Gaynes, B., Lohr, K., Meltzer-Brody, S., Gartlehmer, G. & Swinson, T. (2005) 'Perinatal depression: a systematic review of prevalence and incidence', *Obstetrics & Gynaecology*, 106 (5), pp. 1071-1083.

Holmes, D., Murray, S.J., Perron, A. & Rail, G. (2006) 'Deconstructing the evidence-based discourse in health sciences: truth, power and fascism', *International Journal of Evidence-Based Healthcare*, 4 (3), pp. 180-186.

Ioannidis, J.P.A. (2005) 'Why most published research findings are false', *PLoS Medicine*, 2 (8), pp. 124.

Johnson, R.B., Onwuegbuzie, A.J. & Turner, L.A. (2007) 'Toward a definition of mixed methods research', *Journal of Mixed Methods Research*, 1 (2), pp. 112-133.

Joubert, G. & Ehrlich, R. (2007) *Epidemiology: a research manual for South Africa*. 2nd ed. Cape Town: Oxford University Press Southern Africa.

Last, J.M. (2001) Dictionary of epidemiology. 4th ed. New York: Oxford University Press, p.61.

Maghboeba, M., Simon, C., Van Stade, D. & Buchbinder, M. (2005) 'Community-based participatory research in South Africa: engaging multiple constituents to shape the research question', *Social Science & Medicine*, 61 (12), pp. 2577-2587.

Philipson, T.J. & Jena, A.B. (2005) *Who benefits from new medical technologies? Estimates of consumer and producer surpluses for HIV/ AIDS drugs*. National Bureau for Economic Research.

Popay, J. & Williams, G. (1996) 'Public health research and lay knowledge', *Social Science & Medicine*, 42 (5), pp. 759-768.

Rosenfield, P.L. (1992) 'The potential of transdisciplinary research for sustaining and extending linkages between the health and social sciences', *Social Science & Medicine*, 35 (11), pp. 1343-1357.

Sachs, L. & Kranz, I. (1997) 'Interdisciplinary health research – a symposium', *Social Science & Medicine*, 44 (8), pp. 1209-1210.

Sewankambo, N.K. & Katamba, A. (2009) 'Health systems in Africa: learning from South Africa', *The Lancet*, 374 (9694), pp. 957-959.

U.S. National Library of Medicine (2017) Health statistics. MedlinePlus. Bethesda.

Waraich, P., Goldner, E.M., Somers, J.M. & Hsu, L. (2004) 'Prevalence and incidence of mood disorders: a systematic review of the literature', *The Canadian Journal of Psychiatry*, 49, pp. 124-138.

World Health Organization (2018) Health statistics. Geneva.

Welman, J.C., Kruger, S.J. & Mitchell, B.C. (2005) *Research methodology*. 3rd ed. Cape Town: Oxford University Press Southern Africa.

Chapter 2

Routine Data Sources and Descriptive Epidemiology

The topics of discussion in this chapter are the following:

- Using death certificate data in research
- Types of data, data summaries and correlation
- Demographic, health effect, population-based health data, and the ecological fallacy
- Scenario for calculating standardised mortality ratio

2.1 Using death certificate data in research

DEATH CERTIFICATE DATA can be of value for the purposes of epidemiological research, as epidemiological research helps us to practically make associations between information or data, and the risk factors for disease outcomes in groups or populations. Joubert & Ehrlich (2005) acknowledge that the notion of cause or risk factor could be tricky because most conditions require a number of causes or risk factors working together before the disease outcome could occur. It is important to realize that the validity and reliability of each data element has to be taken into consideration (Bruce et al, 2008).

According to Cohen et al (2007), death certificates contain important information such as age, sex, race, occupation, residential address, date and place of death which could be used in epidemiological studies for the purpose of investigating possible factors associated with breast cancer. The approach would be to identify a country and analyse the death certificate data for a specific period such as from year 2000 to year 2010, and then separate the information by age, sex, occupation, residential address, and place of death. One would conduct a case-control study, and my cases would be all deaths due to breast cancer and my controls would be all deaths other than cancer.

The strengths of death certificate data include its relative ready availability and relative low cost which would make it quicker to interpret the data; and its completeness would allow for interpretation and description of patterns of in-country and cross-country populations (Cohen et al, 2007). The other strength is that death certificate data can be used as a baseline, particularly in states or countries where the use of mammography is not yet well established (Geffken, 2000). Since all types of death are reported on death certificates, it implies that the interpretation of the data would have a lesser probability of being biased.

The limitations of death certificate data include the inconsistencies with which the variables are recorded in different states or countries (Geffken, 2000). Such variations would affect the interpretation of the data in the sense that one would not be able to confidently apply possible factors associated with breast cancer from one country to another country. Another limitation or weakness is the fact that the recording of the cause of death is largely dependent on the physician, because sometimes the physician would just record it as a medical condition instead of being specific. The recording of the cause of death as being a medical condition has somewhat become a norm, particularly in some of the sub-Saharan countries. This implies that using death certificate data to investigate possible factors associated with breast cancer could be a challenge. Hoel et al (1993) highlight the challenge posed by cancer mortality studies because of the issues of quality of the data.

Death certificate data presents a good opportunity to investigate possible factors associated with breast cancer. However, the strengths and limitations need serious consideration as these could have health policy implications.

There are implications of the accuracy or inaccuracy of the death certificate data on research and beyond research. Bruce et al (2008) acknowledge the international variations in the way data is recorded on death certificates. As an extension of this thread, one is curious to find out what is actually recorded on the death certificate in your respective countries or where you are currently based, if the person who has died has been infected with HIV and likely suffered from AIDS?

The foregoing question is being asked because there is on-going debate in parts of sub-Saharan Africa regarding this very point. One group suggests that it should be recorded that the person has died of AIDS, while the second group suggests that the specific disease such as tuberculosis, breast cancer, and pneumonia, among others, should be recoded. As if this was not enough, there is another point of view coming from an ethical angle, which suggests that neither AIDS nor the specific disease should be recorded, but prefers that medical condition or natural causes be recorded instead. The recording of medical condition or natural causes seems to be widespread in the under-resourced public health sector of some of the southern African countries, and this sector caters for the majority of the population (van Rensburg et al, 2008).

A couple of years ago, there was a leading story that flooded the South African media, and this story was about the claim that some doctors in one of the South African provinces were actually recording that patients were suffering from AIDS and therefore died of AIDS. Interestingly, this story raised a huge public outcry in a country that is reeling from the brunt of the epidemic, where it has been reported that

HIV and AIDS are a common denominator for the high mortality, and particularly for the very high maternal mortality and child mortality in South Africa (Pillay, 2008). It is very striking that while South Africa accounts for approximately 0.7 per cent of the world's population, it has more than 17 per cent of the world's new HIV infections (Vecchiatto, 2011).

The other dilemma is that there are people who die at home without having attended any clinic or hospital, and this also raises many questions about what to accurately record on the death certificate. It is interesting to note that it has now become acceptable practice in a number of developed countries to allow terminally ill patients to die at home, and hopefully this does not create issues with recording the correct reason for death (Cohen et al, 2010).

The dilemma of what should be recorded on death certificates poses huge challenges for epidemiological research, and this stifles possible opportunities for intervention, particularly in Southern Africa where the ravages of HIV and AIDS are so brutal.

The mobility of people has increased in recent times. The increase in the mobility of people is possibly fuelled by the fact that the world has now become a global village (Hill, 2009). We see a lot of multinational companies expanding into many corners of the world in a bid to gain a competitive advantage and sometimes in the name of foreign direct investment. As these expansions happen, there is importing and exporting of skills which is accompanied by frequent travels of people from one place to another. Tourism and education are some of the other major reasons why people frequently move from one place to another. What has this got to do with the recording of data on death certificates?

Well, this has much to do with the recording of data on death certificates in the sense that there is a possibility that the diagnosis can be missed if a person who has contracted a disease that is unique to the region where or she comes from, travels to another region where such a disease is not normally known or dealt with. The reality is that that new destination may not even have the tools or tests to confirm that disease. In such an instance, there is a high possibility that a person may be misdiagnosed, and when that person dies there, the wrong diagnosis would very likely be recorded on the death certificate. Cohen et al (2007) emphasise the need for accuracy of information on death certificates to ensure that epidemiological research produces meaningful results that could benefit health systems.

It once happened a few years ago whereby an international tourist who had just visited one of the countries in central Africa fell ill when he arrived in South Africa and was admitted in one of the hospitals in the Gauteng province of South Africa. The person subsequently died within a few days, and it was thought that he had died of other weird causes. The diagnosis of Ebola fever was completely missed despite the battery of tests that were conducted. It was only after a number of the hospital's staff members also fell ill and died showing similar symptoms to the person who had just died that the diagnosis of Ebola fever was finally made. The reason for the misdiagnosis was probably due to the fact that Ebola fever is very rare in South Africa (Nzimande, 1996). The other issue is that misdiagnosis may also be a case of underreporting. Bruce et al (2008) observe that doctors are surprisingly not keen to complete notification forms in most instances of notifiable infectious diseases.

In a nut shell, the mobility of people could contribute to misdiagnoses and recording of the wrong cause of death on death certificates. Misdiagnosis and underreporting can affect the completeness of data recorded on death certificates (Berrino, 2003).

There is prominence of the many variations with regard to the recording of death certificate data. In the midst of these variations and inconsistencies, there is an opportunity and a challenge for epidemiological research. We can still learn something from epidemiological research and we can enhance the opportunity for epidemiological research by ensuring that we pay more attention to the specific research question and by employing the appropriate study design (Bruce et al, 2008).

Evans (2003) mentions some of the study designs commonly used in epidemiology, and these include: cohort, cross-sectional, case control, and randomized control trials. Bruce et al (2008), highlight that we need to be aware of the strengths and weaknesses of each study design to ensure that it is the best for that particular study. Geffken (2000) prefers employing a case-control study to investigate the risk factors associated with breast cancer. It is believed that sometimes, a particular research question could be answered by using more than one study design (Joubert & Ehrlich, 2010).

Having said that, it has to be acknowledged that the best study design, on its own cannot solve the plethora of problems such as misclassification and underreporting which could result in wrong data being recorded on death certificates, as has already been highlighted earlier. In fact, even if the best epidemiological research method is employed, the outcome would not be of great value if the data on death certificates is inaccurate.

In retrospect, there is some positive that we can draw out of epidemiological research in the sense that it can create a stimulus for interventions aimed at addressing the risk factors associated with specific causes of morbidity or mortality in groups or populations. Such stimulus could act as a vehicle to heighten the authorities' focus on the health challenges at hand, thereby creating an opportunity for finding the root cause of the reasons for misdiagnosis or underreporting. If the death certificate data were accurate, it is possible that a pathway or pathways for breast cancer could be hypothesised. Sanderson et al (2006) observe that once a hypothesis has been formed about the pathways for breast cancer, the risk of dying from breast cancer could be influenced. Unfortunately, the disease pathways such as in cancer are not always obvious.

Epidemiological research has a role to play in terms of utilizing death certificate data or any other data source for the purpose of investigating possible factors that are associated with a particular disease. However, epidemiological research could play an even much greater role if the death certificate data were accurate. The reality is that there is great inconsistency and variation in the way death certificate data is recorded and utilised within a country and across countries. This is a much deeper challenge, particularly in many parts of sub-Saharan Africa where there are no clear standards about recording data on death certificates.

2.2 Types of data, data summaries and correlation

TYPES OF DATA

Variable	Type
Age	Continuous
Gender	Categorical
Ethnic group	Categorical
Self-rated health on 5-point scale ('very poor' to 'excellent')	Ranked/ordinal
Height	Continuous
Weight	Continuous
Satisfaction with health care (rated on 10-point scale)	Ranked/ordinal

Summarising data

- Calculating the mean and median for men:

Mean = Sum of scores/Number of scores (Christensen, 2007)

Given sum of scores = 19+30+70+77+46+41+74+53+69+68 = 547

Number of scores = 10

Therefore, the mean = 547/10 = 54.7

According to Joubert & Ehrlich (2007), the median is the 50th percentile or the value which divides the distribution in half whereby the values are arranged from small to large.

Given values arranged from small to large: 19 30 41 46 **53 68** 69 70 74 77

Therefore, the median = (53 + 68)/2 = 60.5

This mean tells us that the average of the distribution is 54.7 and the median tells us that half the distribution falls above 60.5 and half falls below 60.5

We can also see that the median is greater than the mean, which implies that the distribution is left skewed because more than 50 per cent of the distribution is more than the mean (Bruce et al, 2008).

- Calculating the mean and median for women:

Mean = Total of individual scores/Number of scores (Welman et al, 2010)

Given   sum   of   scores   =
94+94+70+63+57+37+71+90+70+60 = 706

Number of scores = 10

Therefore, the mean = 706/10 = 70.6

Median is the midpoint in a distribution, which implies that half the scores fall above the median and half fall below it (Mouton, 2002).

Given values arranged in order: 37 57 60 63 **70 70** 71 90 94 94

Therefore, the median = (70 + 70)/2 = 70

This mean tells us that the average of the distribution is 70.6 and the median tells us that half the distribution falls above 70 and half falls below 70.

We can also see that the median is almost equal to the mean, because there is a difference of only 0.6 which implies that the distribution is almost uniform but very slightly skewed to the right because the mean is only 0.6 more than the median. However, if we do not consider this slight difference of 0.6, we could say the distribution is symmetrical because 50 per cent of the distribution would be more than the mean and the median, and 50 per cent would be less than the mean and the median (Bruce et al, 2008).

Correlation

- From the information in the scatterplot, we can say there is a strong positive relationship between child height and weight.

- Given the correlation coefficient: r = .96

The coefficient of determination = r^2 = $(.96)^2$ = .92

This implies that 92 per cent of the total variation in weight is explained by the variation in height. However, there is still a remainder of 8 per cent of the variation which may not be easily explained because it may be due to unknown factors (Bruce et al, 2008).

2.3 Demographic, health effect, population-based health data, and the ecological fallacy

THE ISSUE OF INFLUENZA vaccinations really needs serious attention, as some of the research studies have highlighted that the influenza vaccine does not confer protection to approximately 42 per cent of the studied population. Of course, we may not draw conclusions based on one study or a few studies, but the fact that some people got sick after the vaccinations were administered is an issue, nevertheless. In such cases, it makes it even more important for us to pay particular attention to the weaknesses of our research studies to ensure that we do not put people at risk at the cost of research. Although some researchers indicate that influenza vaccinations are very crucial for people that are deemed to be vulnerable, such as children and the elderly, other researchers report that the effectiveness of these vaccinations has not been convincing (Katz, 1987). Talbot et al (2010), add that currently, there is controversy about the immunogenicity of seasonal trivalent influenza vaccine in certain populations.

Given this situation, one wonders if the consistent worldwide recommendation to vaccinate people, particularly those that are deemed vulnerable such as children and the elderly is a fallacy (Rida et al, 2011). An observation is that the controversies take different forms in different contexts (Lantos et al, 2010). In the more affluent areas such as in the developed countries, parents tend to have fears about negative consequences of the vaccinations on their children, whereas in the rural areas where the majority of the people live, parents tend not to have many questions.

A couple of years ago, it once happened that there was a massive project in collaboration with an international health/development agency to administer an anti-helminth vaccine on all primary school children in one of the southern African countries. The first phase of the project yielded dire results as many of the vaccinated children fell ill and had to be admitted into hospitals and a few of them were subsequently reported to have died as a result of the anti-helminth vaccine. This was a big story in the local media, and parents were also raising their disapproval of such mass immunization as the immunization was done while the children were at school. The government of that particular country acted quickly, and ordered that the immunization be stopped with immediate effect.

What one is trying to highlight from that southern African country's story is that an ecological study was probably done, and this might have indicated that the country's children were at high risk of helminth infections. However, it was probably a fallacy because it assumed that all individual children of that country shared the same risk and characteristics. Sabatelli et al (2008), highlight that the dynamics of infections are very complex as they may be influenced by many factors arising from a variety of exposures and immunity-related factors. Therefore, the unique variations in different places should be taken into account (Bruce et al, 2008).

A colleague highlighted the issue of polio in Nigeria and the vulnerability of children who live in low-socioeconomic settings. It is possible that the broad-brush global immunisation of all children under the age of five against polio is a fallacy. It has now been discovered that after all these many years of polio immunisation, the OPV carries some risk in the sense that it is excreted and can circulate in the environment and thereby result in vaccine derived polio virus (vDPV) or a wild type of polio virus (Davies, 2013). Although there have only been approximately 114 virologically confirmed vaccine derived polio cases worldwide thus far, it is one too many (Davies, 2013).

At least the World Health Organisation has acknowledged the risk of vaccine derived polio virus, and has advised that a combination of the oral polio vaccine (OPV) and the inactivated polio vaccine (IPV) be used in the interim, with the aim of phasing out the OPV in the next couple of years. Since the IPV is more expensive than the OPV, the cost implications will be a challenge for many countries, particularly developing countries as this combination of OPV/IPV will cost much more. If it cost $600 000 for the project to administer an OPV to 650 000 children in Madagascar between August 2005 and October 2005, one can imagine the cost implications of the OPV/IPV combination (UNICEF, 2005). The draft Polio Eradication and Endgame Strategic Plan (2013-2018) suggests that at least one dose of IPV should be universally adopted as part of routine immunization by 2015 (Polio Eradication Initiative, 2013).

Although Nigeria is the only polio-endemic country in Africa, the eradication of polio still remains an imperative for all African countries (Cooke, 2012). It is encouraging to see that this imperative has been shown by African governments' resolution through the African Regional Committee declaring that the persistence of polio is a national public health emergency (Kakujaha, 2011). This implies that all African countries should scale up their efforts in ensuring that polio is eradicated. I say this because there have been at least ten African countries that have reported cases of polio during the past few years, and it has been shown that these have generally been cases of imported polio (UNICEF, 2011).

Much as we have seen that there has been a declaration by the African Regional Committee for the eradication of polio, we need to bear in mind that high level political endorsement does not always translate into effective implementation on the ground. Well, perhaps, the high level political endorsement on immunization is also a fallacy. Nevertheless, it has to be acknowledged that immunisations are one of the greatest public health achievements of the 20th century (Vangjel, 2011).

It would be interesting to conduct an ecological study with particular focus on assessing readily available data, on the aggregated mean blood pressure of shift workers in the agricultural, manufacturing and mining sectors of southern African countries such as the Kingdom of Swaziland (Eswatini), Republic of South Africa, Botswana and Namibia, among others. The 'healthy worker effect' will certainly be taken into consideration as this data will only be focused on employees and not the general public. In fact, the 'healthy worker effect' could be one of the reasons the blood pressure means may be underreported in some instances, as highlighted earlier.

If this ecological study indicates a strong association between shift-work and high blood pressure, it may be tempting to conclude that it is a causal association (Bruce et al, 2008). It may also be tempting to stretch this association to other cardiovascular disorders. For that reason, the title of the study below should have been more specific to high blood pressure rather than cardiovascular disorders as a whole because there is a plethora of cardiovascular disorders that may not necessarily be linked to high blood pressure. Be as it may, the ecological study could enable us to generate a hypothesis about the association or no association between shift-work and high blood pressure. This could then be investigated further through more specific and in-depth study designs to see if there is a causal effect or no causal effect at an individual level. If the more specific studies find no causal association between shift-work and high blood pressure at individual level and yet the ecological study showed a strong association, it implies that this could be an ecological fallacy.

Further studies could also help us to identify possible other factors that could influence the causal association between shift-work and high blood pressure at individual level, if there is any at all. In other words this tells us that an ecological study can pave the way for more in-depth investigations about causal relationships between variables. However, this does not by any means imply that the in-depth studies do not have their own limitations. Since this study will be an international study, some researchers highlight that confounding is more pronounced in international studies, and this could be a major weakness as countries sometimes differ markedly in many aspects (Althabe et al, 2006).

Moreover, given the migration of workforce within the Southern Africa region, it is possible that the sectors of focus in this study will have varying degrees of heterogeneity which could influence the data. Pickett & Pearl (2001) highlight that the bigger the degree of heterogeneity, the bigger the margin of error.

CARDIOVASCULAR DISORDERS among shift workers: an ecological study of Southern African countries

Introduction:

The health effects of shift work have been an issue of debate among researchers. There is paucity of studies on the health effects of shift work among industrial workers in Southern Africa. The majority of shift workers in the agricultural, manufacturing and mining sectors of Southern Africa are blue collar and they come from low socio-economic backgrounds (Naidoo, 2009). Sub-Saharan Africa is now faced with an epidemic of non-communicable diseases such as high blood pressure (Mayosi et al, 2009). There is a possibility that shift work causes cardiovascular disorders (LaDou, 2007). The objective of this ecological study is to test the hypothesis that shift work causes high blood pressure among shift workers.

Methodology:

The cross-sectional ecological study design, will involve an assessment of annual occupational health reports of the agricultural, manufacturing and mining sectors of the Kingdom of Swaziland (Eswatini), Republic of South Africa, Botswana, and Namibia, to determine the mean blood pressure of shift workers in the respective industries. The annual occupational health reports to be assessed will be for the period 2010 to 2013.

Discussion:

The ecological fallacy might influence one's interpretation of the study results in the sense that these results will not be a true reflection of each individual represented by the mean blood pressure data in this study (Pickett et al, 2005). There is a possibility that there are other confounding factors that might be uniquely collateral or contralateral for the health outcome of blood pressure for each individual despite the similar exposure which in this case is shift work (Macinko, et al, 2003). Genetic factors may come into play as well as individuals have different predispositions to cardiovascular disorders such as high blood pressure than others. It is also important to consider that some of the employees in the industries of focus in this study may have migrated from other countries, and as a result, their predisposition may also be unique. Schwartz (1994) observes that there is complexity of the interplay of aetiological factors of any particular disease.

Moreover, the shift pattern may differ from industry to industry and from country to country, which implies that it would not be proper to conclude with certainty about whether shift work has direct effect on an individual's blood pressure or not. Bruce et al (2008) observe that sources of data do not provide the full picture.

The 'healthy worker effect' cannot be ruled out, because it is possible that there could be underreporting of the mean blood pressure as sickly workers with uncontrolled high blood pressure or with complications from high blood pressure may have been taken out of service or boarded off. Pearce (2000) argues that much as we have to be aware of the 'ecological fallacy' we also need to be careful of the 'individualistic fallacy'.

Conclusion:

An ecological study can be useful as a quick 'scan' to give us an idea about a possible association between an exposure and a health outcome in populations (Pearce, 2000). However, such a study has its limitations as it is prone to the ecological fallacy which assumes that all the employees of the industries that were assessed in this study share the social and health characteristics of that area.

2.4 Scenario for calculating standardised mortality ratio

STANDARDISATION

- Prior to 31 March 2013, and going as far back as 2001, there existed a number of Primary Care Trusts (PCTs) as part of the National Health Service (NHS) in England. Up to 2011, these PCTs provided community services directly, and their total budget was approximately 80 per cent of the total NHS budget. As such, the PCTs served a sizable population. However, it was not appropriate to compare the crude mortality rates within the PCT population with those for England and Wales because this could have been influenced by the difference in age distribution between the PCT population and that of England and Wales. For example, it may happen that the PCT population in Bolton had a much higher proportion of older people compared to other PCTs, and this could be masked if we compared with the age proportions of England and Wales, in general. Joubert & Ehrlich (2010) report that older age groups tend to have a higher mortality rate compared to younger age groups.

- Calculation of a standardized mortality ratio (SMR) makes it appropriate to compare mortality rates in this situation because the SMR takes account of the differences in age distribution of the PCT population and that of Wales and England. Heijink et al (2008) report that calculating a standardized mortality ratio compensates for the differences in the distribution mix.
- The SMR is an indirect form of standardization
- Calculation of the expected deaths for the Bolton PCT:

According to Joubert & Ehrlich (2010), the expected deaths for a specific age group in specific population can be calculated by multiplying the age-specific death rate of standard population by the population size of matching age category of the population of interest. Adding these can then give the 'expected deaths' of the population of interest (Bruce et al, 2008)

Based on the above explanation and the given table below, we can calculate the 'expected deaths' in Bolton PCT as follows:

'Expected deaths' for age group (0-4) = 1.61/1000 x 950 = 1.53

'Expected deaths for age group (15-24) = 0.98/1000 x 724 = 0.71

'Expected deaths for age group (25-44) = 2.32/1000 x 932 = 2.16

'Expected deaths for age group (45-64) = 13.64/1000 x 870 = 11.87

'Expected deaths for age group (65-84) = 64.45/1000 x 423 = 27.26

'Expected deaths for age group (85+) = 187.13/1000 x 24 = 4.49

Therefore,

Expected deaths for the Bolton PCT = 1.53 + 0.71 + 2.16 + 11.87 + 27.26 + 4.49 = **48.02**

Age group	Deaths in Bolton PCT	Bolton PCT population	England and Wales mortality rate (per 1,000/year)	Deaths 'expected' in Bolton PCT
0-14	2	950	1.61	1.53
15-24	1	724	0.98	0.71
25-44	5	932	2.32	2.16
45-64	12	870	13.64	11.87
65-84	26	423	64.45	27.26
85+	8	24	187.13	4.49
Total	54	3,923	12.41	**48.02**

- According to Bruce et al (2008),

SMR = Total number of observed deaths / Total number of expected deaths

Therefore, SMR for the Bolton PCT = 54 / 48.02 = 1.12

It is noteworthy that the reference SMR is usually expressed as 100 (Brown & Barraclough, 2000). This implies that the SMR for the Bolton PCT can be expressed as 1.12 x 100 = **112**

Based on the SMR for the Bolton PCT, it can be interpreted that independent of the influence of age distribution, the SMR for the Bolton PCT is 12 per cent higher than that of England and Wales (Bruce et al, 2008).

- Calculating and interpreting the confidence interval for the SMR:

Upper limit of 95% CI for SMR = 112 + [1.96 x (112/ square root of 54)]

= 141.873

Lower limit of 95% CI for SMR = 112 – [1.96 X (112 / square root of 54)]

= 82.127

We can say that the Bolton PCT SMR is 112, with a 95 per cent confidence interval of 82 – 142. This implies that we can be 95 per cent certain that the true SMR for the Bolton PCT lies between 82 and 142, or 18 per cent below and 41 per cent above the England and Wales' level of mortality (Bruce et al, 2008). The confidence interval of 82 – 142 is wide. Maree (2010) highlights that there is a higher level of confidence if the confidence interval is wider, and there is a lower level of confidence if the confidence interval is narrower. In this case, we can say we have a higher level of confidence that the true SMR for the Bolton PCT lies between 82 and 142.

REFERENCES

Berrino, F. (2003) 'The EUROCARE study: strengths, limitations and perspectives of population-based, comparative survival studies', *Annals of Oncology*, 14 (5), pp. v9-v13.

Brown, S. & Barraclough, B. (2000) 'Causes of the excess mortality of schizophrenia', *The British Journal of Psychiatry*, 177, pp. 212-217.

Bruce, N., Pope, D. & Stanistreet, D. (2008) 'Routine data sources and descriptive epidemiology'. In: *Quantitative research methods for health research: a practical guide to epidemiology*. Chichester: John Wiley & Sons, Ltd.

Christensen, L.B. (2007) 'Data analysis'. In: *Experimental methodology*. 10th ed. Boston: Pearson.

Cohen, J., Houttekier, D., Onwuteaka-Philipsen, B., Miccinesi, G., Addington-Hall, J., Kaasa, S., Bilsen, J. & Deliens, L. (2010) 'Which patients with cancer die at home? A study of six European countries using death certificate data', *Journal of Clinical Oncology*, 28 (13), pp. 2267-2273.

Cohen, J., Bilsen, J., Missinesi, G., Lofmark, R., Addington-Hall, J., Kaasa, S., Norup, M.,Van der Wal, G. & Deliens, L. (2007) 'Using death certificate data to study place of death in 9 European countries: opportunities and weaknesses', *BioMed Central Public Health*, 7, pp. 283-292.

Cooke, J.G. (2012) *Polio in Nigeria*. Centre for Strategic and International Studies [Online]. Available from: http://www.csis.org

Evans, D. (2003) 'Hierarchy of evidence: a framework for ranking evidence evaluating healthcare interventions', *Journal of Clinical Nursing*, 12, pp. 77-84.

Davies, R. (2013) 'Inactivated polio vaccine: its proposed role in the final stages of polio eradication', *The Pan African Medical Journal*, 14, p. 112.

Geffken, D.F. , Perry, M.J. & Callas, P.W. (2000) 'Association of occupation and breast cancer mortality in the state of Vermont, 1989-1993', *Massachusetts Journal of Medicine*, 5, pp. 75-79.

Heijink, R., Koolman, X., Pieter, D., Van der Veen, A., Jarman, B. & Westert, G. (2008) 'Measuring and explaining mortality in Dutch hospitals: the hospital standardization mortality rate between 2003 and 2005', *BMC Health Services Research*, 8, p. 73.

Hill, C.W.L. (2009) *International business: competing in the global marketplace.* 7th ed. Boston: McGraw-Hill International Edition.

Hoel, D.G., Ron, E., Carter, R. & Mabuchi, K. (1993) 'Influence of death certificate errors on cancer mortality trends', *Journal of the National Cancer Institute*, 85 (13), pp. 1063-1068

Joubert, G. & Ehrlich, R. (2007) *Epidemiology: a research manual for South Africa.* 2nd ed. Cape Town: Oxford University Press Southern Africa.

Kakujaha, A. (2011) 'Polio: much done, much still to be done', *The Southern Times*, 11 November.

Katz, S.L. (1987) Controversies in immunisation', *Pediatric Infectious Disease Journal*, 6 (6), pp. 607-613.

LaDou, J. (2007) Stress at work. In: *Occupational & environmental medicine.* New York: McGraw-Hill.

Lantos, J.D. Jackson, M.A., Opel, D.J., Maree, M. & Myers, A., Connelly, B.L. (2010) 'Controversies in vaccine mandates', *Current Problems in Pediatric and Adolescent Health Care*, 40 (3), pp. 38-58.

Macinko, J., Starfield, B. & Shi, L. (2003) 'The contribution of primary care systems to health outcomes within organisation for economic cooperation and development (OECD) countries, 1970-1998', *Health Services Research*, 35 (3), pp. 831-865.

Maree, K. (2010) 'Statistical analysis II: inferential statistics'. In: *First steps in research*. Pretoria: Van Schaik.

Mayosi, B.M., Flisher, A.J., Lalloo, U.G., Sitas, F., Tollman, S.M. & Bradshaw, D. (2009) 'The burden of non-communicable diseases in South Africa', *The Lancet*, 374(9693), pp. 934-947.

Mouton, J. (2002) 'Data analysis and interpretation'. In: *Understanding social research*. Pretoria: Van Schaik.

Naidoo, R. (2009) 'The work and health in Southern Africa (WAHSA) programme – overall experience and the way forward', *Occupational Health Southern Africa*, 15, pp. 2-6.

Nzimande, P.N. (1996) *Communicable in the African continent*. 2nd ed. Pinetown: Alberts Publishers.

Pearce, N. (2000) 'The ecological fallacy strikes back', *Journal of Epidemiology & Community Health*, 54, pp. 326-327.

Pickett, K.E., Kelly, S., Brunner, E., Lobstein, T. & Wilkinson, R.G. (2005) 'Wider income gaps, wider waistbands? An ecological study of obesity and income inequality', *Journal of Epidemiology & Community Health*, 59 (8), pp. 670-674.

Pillay, R. (208) 'Managerial competencies of hospital managers in South Africa: a survey of managers in the public and private sectors', *Human Resources for Health*, 6 (4), pp. 1-7.

Polio Eradication Initiative (2013) *Polio eradication and endgame strategic plan (2013-2018)*.

Sabatelli, L, Ghani, A.C., Rodrigues, L.C., Hotez, P.J. & Brooker, S. (2008) 'Modelling heterogeneity and the impact of chemotherapy and vaccination against human hookworm', *Journal of the Royal Society Interface*, 5 (28): pp. 1329-134.

Sanderson, M., Daling, J.R., Doody, D.R. & Malone, K.E. (2006) 'Perinatal factors and mortality from breast cancer', *Cancer Epidemiology, Biomarkers & Prevention*, 15, pp. 1984-1987.

Schwartz, S. (1994) 'The fallacy of the ecological fallacy', *American Journal of Public Health*, 84 (5), pp. 819-824.

Talbot, H.K., Rock, M.T., Johnson, C., Tussey, L., Karita, U., Shanker, A., Shaw, A.R. & Taylor, D.N. (2010) 'Trivalent influenza vaccine when given with vax102, a recombinant influenza m2e fused to the tlr5 ligand flagellin', *PLoS ONE*, 5 (12), pp. 1-7.

UNICEF (2011) *Polio eradication in Eastern and Southern Africa.* Available from: http://www.unicef.org/esaro/5479_polio.html

Vangjel, L. (2011) '*The economics of child health*', Humanities and Social Sciences, 72 (2-A): p. 686.

Van Rensburg, D.H.C.J., Steyn, F., Schneider, H. & Loffstadt, L. (2008) 'Human resource development and antiretroviral treatment in Free State province, South Africa', *Human Resources for Health*, 6 (15), pp. 1-10.

Vecchiatto, P. (2011) *Current health system not sustainable.* Available from: http://www.businesslive.co.za/southafrica/2011/06/29/current-health-system-unsustainable

Welman, C., Kruger, F. & Mitchell, B. (2010) 'Data analysis and interpretation of results'. In: *Research methodology.* Cape Town: Oxford University Press.

Chapter 3

Surveys

This chapter covers the following topics:

- Survey design
- Methods of sampling

3.1 Survey design

IMAGINE A RESEARCHERS' population of interest being all the people who live in Aigburth (a suburb of Liverpool). The first step would be to have a sampling frame which includes the characteristics of the sample such as the name and surnames, contact details, addresses, telephone numbers. The sampling frame could be obtained from a number of sources such as telephone directory, municipality register, or even lists from general practitioners in that suburb. Although it is the ideal to get the list of the entire population of Aigburth, but we have to realize that the sampling frame may not contain the list of every person in that suburb.

The method of sampling that could be used is simple random sampling, whereby each person on the list will be given a specific code such as A1, A2, and so on. Suppose the researchers want to choose 1000 out of a total of 5 000 people in the sample frame, then 5000 codes will be randomly selected for example by using a computer programme. It has to be borne in mind that simple random sampling is dependent on chance. This means that, if we are lucky, we may get a sample that is a true representation of the population of interest, but if we are not lucky, the sample may not be a true representation of the population of interest. It is worth noting that a sampling error may occur if different random samples of the same size such as 1000 from the same sample frame give different means which may also differ from the mean of the population of interest.

Once the researchers have confirmed the randomly selected sample from the sampling frame, they should conduct a survey through the use of questionnaires so that they could estimate the proportion of people in Aigburth who regularly smoke. Before the survey is conducted, it would be important to make the participants aware about the research survey, in advance, and this should be clearly explained to them so that they are prepared. The questionnaires with a cover letter can then be mailed to the individuals' addresses. The cover letter should clearly explain what the survey is all about and the deadline for submitting the completed questionnaires should be clearly indicated. It is possible that not all questionnaires will be completed or returned due to reasons such as inability, relocation, among others.

The implications of the sample size are that there could be a possible underrepresentation of the population and an overrepresentation of the population. It is therefore important to calculate the sample size with some degree of precision to ensure that there is accuracy in the sample mean which should reflect a true picture of the population of interest. In this regard, the researchers may need to calculate the standard error and the 95 per cent confidence interval to estimate the proportion of people who regularly smoke to within a specified level of error.

It is generally believed that a larger sample size provides a better chance to yield information or results that could be generalised to the population of interest. It is indeed good to have a large sample size especially when we study larger populations (Maree, 2010). However, it may happen that the sample size could be unnecessarily large, and this could create many problems in terms of the collection and analysis of the large amounts of data and unnecessary costs could also be incurred. Joubert & Ehrlich (2007) observe that sometimes when we study larger populations it is a matter of knowing how large the sample size should be. Bearing that it in mind, it would probably be a better idea to involve a statistician to assist with calculating an ideal sample size and make the necessary adjustments according to the sampling method that we have chosen (Bruce et al, 2008). Such adjustments could indicate the design effect of the sampling method and this indicates how the sampling design influences the accuracy of the estimates (Joubert & Ehrlich (2007).

Some studies highlight that the sample size does not necessarily have to be large when a stratified sampling method is employed, and yet stratified sampling has a better chance of having a more representative sample than simple random sampling (Welman et al, 2005). To illustrate this point, suppose there is a total population of 5000 at Aigburth (a suburb of Liverpool) and the researchers wish to investigate the proportion of people who regularly smoke in that suburb. If the researchers decide to use simple random sampling, they may need to study a larger proportion of the population such as 1000 people. It may happen that the selected sample of 1000 randomly selected people predominantly comprises one segment of the population, and certain segments of the population may not be represented at all.

However, if the researchers prefer to use stratified sampling, they will have to ensure that at least all strata of the population are included (Welman et al, 2005). In other words, the researchers will ensure that they randomly select a similar percentage of people from each stratum of the population. In this regard, the different strata of the population of Aigburth could be the different age categories or the different sexes or the different ethnic groups.

As part of our self-care programme, we will possibly consider employing a stratified sampling method to estimate the proportion of people who regularly drink alcohol in different countries of Southern Africa. Cost implications and the amount of time required to conduct such a study will influence one's choice of the study design as well. Johnson et al (2001) observe that the willingness to participate and honesty with regard to how the respondents respond in a survey is another important factor that can influence the accuracy of the information to be analysed.

In survey research, the intention is to have accurate information that is representative of the population of interest (Bruce et al, 2008). However, getting accurate information that is representative of the population of interest has become one of the biggest challenges facing researchers. It is a truism that "one of the interesting things about an intended random sample is that those who actually return the questionnaires may not end up being a random sample" (Holmes, 2013). This indicates that researchers have to come up with ways of dealing with this problem.

Interestingly, some researchers have proposed various creative ways of dealing with this problem, but some of these various ways have not been effective in all settings. Grava-Gubins & Scott (2008) observe that conducting surveys among professionals remains problematic because the response rate does not improve even after implementing various creative ways such as shortening the survey, providing incentives, making follow-ups and creative marketing.

Some researchers report that employing a tailored design method yields positive results because it improves response rate in postal surveys (Thorpe et al, 2008). It is highlighted that the tailored design method involves key elements such as: personalized correspondence; using a respondent-friendly questionnaire; using return envelopes with first class registered mail; financial incentives; and special follow up contact by certified mail or telephone call (Scott et al, 2011). This could possibly work for populations that are in the developed countries and possibly also in the urban areas of developing countries, because the majority of people who live in developing countries such as in Southern Africa, are in the rural areas where mail correspondence could be a challenge. VanGeest et al (2007) report that the response rate among professionals increases if the survey research is endorsed by a professional body or association. Some studies indicate that surveys that have a focused participatory approach with incentives for participating show better response rates especially among the youth (Claudio & Stingone, 2008).

This highlights the importance of ensuring that a survey research should be tailor made for that particular population of interest as settings always have many variations in terms of demographics, culture and norms. In that regard, I do not think there is a standard way of dealing with the problem. For example, in many parts of Southern Africa, it would be crucial to get buy-in from the chiefs or councillors of that particular area of focus, before the survey research is even started. The chiefs and councillors are very influential in their respective communities, and once they have endorsed the idea of a proposed survey research, there is a better chance for a good response rate. A good response rate gives a better chance for a representative sample and accuracy of information, and minimizes the chance of a sampling bias.

Imagine a study aimed at measuring the prevalence of insomnia among the working population of the industrial city of uMhlathuze in the north east coast of the South African province of KwaZulu-Natal. The sampling frame would be obtained from the employee registers of all the different industries of the city of uMhlathuze. Stratified probability sampling would be employed, and the stratification would be based on age, sex, occupation, shift pattern, industry, and length of service. Joubert & Ehrlich (2007) observe that stratified probability sampling is easy to apply where full lists such as employee registers can be obtained.

An advance letter would be issued to all potential respondents explaining the purpose of the survey, explaining that participants would be selected at random, that participation would be voluntary, and that confidentiality would be maintained and guaranteed (Roth et al, 2011). The advance letter would also explain that participation in the survey would not affect the participants' employment, that participants would be free to opt out of the survey at any time or they could phone a specified toll-free number for further information, and that there would be a financial incentive for participating in the survey (Scott et al, 2011).

Consent would first be obtained from each participant before telephonic interviews are conducted (Roth et al, 2011). The telephonic interviews would be based on a brief insomnia questionnaire which would be a condensed hybrid of the World Health Organisation's International Statistical Classification of Diseases, Research Diagnostic Criteria for insomnia, International Classification of Sleep Disorders, and the DSM-IV-TR criteria (Roth et al, 2011). It is critical to pay attention to the question type, length of the questions, ordering of the questions, phrasing and structure of the questions (Bruce et al, 2008).

It is possible that some of the people randomly selected to participate in the survey may not contribute to the research, and this may negatively affect the response rate and the representativity of the population of interest. According to Bruce et al (2008), such people may include those that cannot be contacted and those that decline to participate in the survey. Sturgis et al (2006), highlight that the response rate in a survey is usually strongly linked to the characteristics of the environment of focus. Mosavel et al (2005) observe that the

South African population is very sensitive, and research surveys are usually met with suspicion from different angles, and in particular from a politico-socio-economic angle. The sensitivity of communities to research surveys is not unique to South Africa, but is a global issue, and the only difference is the magnitude of that sensitiveness.

We may need to come up with ways of gaining the trust of the population of focus in the industrial city of uMhlathuze, in order not to risk the possibility of a high non-response bias. It is recommended that stratum-specific results be proportionately weighted before the overall results can be analysed (Joubert & Ehrlich, 2007). It is worth mentioning that telephonic surveys can be tricky as any slight tension during the interview may lead to outright refusals (O'Rourke & Blair, 1983). In that vein, it is recommended that there be expertise in the planning, execution and analysis stages of such survey research to prevent or minimize non response bias (Draugalis & Plaza, 2009).

3.2 Methods of sampling

STRATIFIED RANDOM SAMPLING is indeed a good choice to make because it has two key advantages, including the fact there is a higher probability of a representative sample and that it requires a smaller sample size compared to simple random sampling (Welman et al, 2005). However, it is very important to ensure that stratum-specific results are proportionately adjusted or weighted when combining them especially if strata are not chosen proportionately to their size in the study population (Joubert & Ehrlich, 2007). It is considered that a constant sample fraction may be used to increase the level of precision in the sample estimate when a stratified sampling method is employed (Bruce et al, 2008).

The importance of ensuring that the researchers have a clear understanding of the composition of the population of interest, before the survey is even carried out, is of importance. It may happen that the sampling frame could be wrongly finalized, with the understanding that the demographic records of the entire geographical area of interest are complete, only to find that there is or are groups of people or strata that have been unwittingly excluded. There are a number of reasons why certain groups of people could be unwittingly excluded from the sample frame. These reasons may include: homelessness, illiteracy, living in informal settlements, and other various forms of social exclusion or marginalization. Igboamalu & Govender (2013) observe that illiteracy and low socioeconomic status have a huge bearing on low response rates in research surveys.

A typical example is that of South Africa where there are so many people living in informal settlements in the peri-urban areas and most of these people frequently migrate from one place to another in search for jobs. Another example is that of the indigenous minority groups such as the San of Southern Africa some of whom still lead a semi-nomadic life, and their language of communication is marginalized and not well understood in the mainstream (Ohenjo et al, 2006). In this regard, if we were to conduct a stratified random sampling based on demographic information obtained from municipality registers or telephone directories, a lot of the people who do not appear on the records could be missed. As a result this could lead to sampling error, even though sampling error is thought to be reduced in stratified random sampling compared to simple random sampling (Bruce et al, 2008).

It is suggested that a specific sampling method such as snowball sampling be employed in the case of challenges such as when dealing with people that are very difficult to reach (Bruce et al, 2008). It can be concluded that the different sampling methods have their advantages and disadvantages. It is therefore advisable that the research team choose a sampling method that is suitable for a specific situation or circumstance to ensure accuracy of data and analysis, and representativeness of the population of interest (Maree, 2010).

In survey work we use samples because it may not be possible to study the whole population (Joubert & Ehrlich, 2007). The sample should be a true representation of the population in which we want to base our research on (Grava-Gubins & Scott, 2008). For example, imagine the suburb of Aigburth has a population of 50 000 and we want to estimate the number of people who regularly smoke in that particular suburb. Using samples may not require that we study each and every individual in that suburb, but a portion of the population can be selected, and as long as the selected sample is representative of the general population of Aigburth, the number of people who regularly smoke can be estimated.

Selection bias means that we systematically choose a sample that is an underrepresentation or an overrepresentation of the population that we want to study (Bruce et al, 2008). In that case, it means that we cannot infer the results we get from the selected sample to the general population of interest. For example, a selection bias may occur if the selected sample differs from the general population of interest (Woolf et al, 2000).

Random sampling overcomes selection bias because in random sampling the selection of the sample is purely based on chance (Bruce et al, 2008). In random sampling, there is generally no subjective preference of a specific group in the population of interest. Although it cannot be ruled out that there is a chance that the randomly chosen sample may not be representative of the general population, but such a probability is small compared to when a non-random sampling is employed. Robins et al (2000) observe that the selection bias on un-observables nor its magnitude is minimized if random sampling is employed in survey research.

A sampling frame is a list that contains the full details of the individuals that we want to study in that population (Bruce et al, 2013). Whittmore & Knafl (2005) defines a sampling frame as the list of units to be studied. An example of a sampling frame is all the residents of a particular town whose details can be obtained from a voters register. The details on the voters register may contain the name, surname, date of birth, physical address, postal address, and telephone number of each resident who qualifies for inclusion in the survey research (Thorpe et al, 2008).

Standard error and confidence interval for population mean:

Standard error = s / square root of n

Given, n = 300

Given, s = 10.5

Therefore, standard error = 300 / square root of 52.3 = 1.45

95 per cent confidence interval around the sample mean:

(Mean − 1.96s / square root of n, mean + 1.96s / square root of n)

(52.3 − 1.96 x 10.5 / square root of 300, 52.3 + 1.96 x 10.5 / square root of 300)

Therefore 95 per cent confidence interval around the mean is (51.1, 53.5)

This implies that we are 95 per cent confident that the mean body weight of secondary school children lies between 51.1 kg and 53.5 kg.

It is true that stratification is usually employed for a specific reason. It is reported that stratification can be specifically employed to deal with confounding in the study design, in the analysis, or in both (Bruce et al, 2013). Confounding occurs when the exposed and non-exposed groups in the population of interest are not comparable due to inherent differences in background disease risk, usually due to exposure to other risk factors or extraneous factors (Cromar et al, 2006).

Suppose the aim of our research was to see if there is an association between shift work and insomnia among the working population of the industrial town of uMhlathuze in the South African province of KwaZulu-Natal. It is possible that we may get results indicating that not all the workers who were exposed to the same shift work, suffer from insomnia. The health outcome may not be a direct result of shift work, but it could also be influenced by other factors such as age, sex, smoking, alcohol consumption, and other inherent predispositions to insomnia.

In our study design, if we suspect alcohol consumption to be a confounding factor, we could stratify on alcohol consumption by dividing the population of interest into alcohol consumers and non-alcohol consumers, and we could select a specified proportion of cases and controls from each stratum (Bruce et al, 2008). It is highlighted that it is also possible to carry out post-stratification or stratification during the analysis of results even if the sample was not stratified, provided information on the extraneous factors was collected (Bruce et al, 2013). However, the challenge with post-stratification is that it cannot be guaranteed that there would be enough cases and controls in the different strata (Bruce et al, 2013). Nonetheless, by using a stratified analysis, the researcher attempts to adjust for, or remove the effect of, an extraneous factor which is related to the exposure and the health outcome (Joubert & Ehrlich, 2007).

Stratification is usually employed for a specific reason of eliminating confounding such as in case control studies (Bruce et al, 2008). Confounding elements could be used in the broad sense to include researcher, participant and context effects, and these pose a threat to the reliability of data collected (Mouton, 2002). It is therefore important to control for extraneous factors or confounding factors in order to attain internal validity (Christensen, 2007).

It is acknowledged that using stratification with more than two variables, may result in the sample getting smaller and smaller. It can be observed that having a shrinking sample could increase the chance of sampling bias. In that case, simple random sampling could be preferred.

However, it is also possible that using simple random sampling could result in a non-representative sample as those randomly selected could end up not being a random sample due to the likelihood of self-selection (Draugalis & Plaza, 2009). At the same time, since the sampling frame of the working population of the industrial city of uMhlathuze is so huge, simple random sampling could require a larger sample which could be very difficult to manage especially in the circumstance of budget constraints (Welman et al, 2005). It is interesting to note that some researchers report that smaller samples may not necessarily represent sampling bias, but what matters the most in survey research is the quality of how the sample is selected, and how the data is collected and analysed and to ensure that it is representative of the population of interest (McCarty, 2003).

In that regard, it is therefore tempting to use stratification, because in stratification we do not necessarily have to deal with a larger sample and we can also use a constant sampling fraction to increase the precision of our sampling estimate unlike in simple random sampling (Joubert & Ehrlich, 2007). Of course, it does make a lot of sense to stick to one variable or two variables when a stratified probability sampling is employed as this could help us avoid the risk of a shrinking sample size as when using more variables. Sticking to one variable such as shift pattern will also make it easier for us to manage in terms of analysis of the results as opposed to when more variables were involved. Bruce et al (2008) add that using stratified probability sampling is an advantage over using simple random sampling because stratification gives a better chance of a representative sample and can yield more reliable results.

Simple random sampling is preferred when more than two variables are used, and stratified probability sampling could be employed when a maximum of one or two variables is used. Variables such as age, sex, occupation or social class could still assist us in terms of assessing non-response bias, to see if there is a match between the responders and non-responders in the population of interest (Bruce et al, 2008).

The issue of antenatal care and perinatal outcomes is pertinent in every country, and, particularly so in sub-Saharan Africa, as this region is faced with a huge burden of disease, high crude birth rates, and also very high maternal and infant mortality rates (de Haan, 2005). Studies highlight that the maternal and infant morbidity and mortality issues are so serious in sub-Saharan Africa that such issues threaten to overwhelm the already weak health systems and have undermined the potential of this region to meet most of the targets of the Millennium Development Goals (Chopra, 2009). As such, if these issues are not addressed with a sense of urgency through effective leadership, achievement of the Sustainable Development Goals will also be a challenge.

Be as it may, we cannot afford to lose any hope because through epidemiological research, we can get an idea of the magnitude of possible associations with the health outcomes so that interventions could be implemented (Bruce et al, 2008). One such glimmer of hope was the then proposed cohort survey to explore the associations between background and behavioural decisions on antenatal care attendance and perinatal outcomes in Kenya. It was interesting to note that in the cohort survey, the plan was to recruit some people from the same communities where the research would be conducted so that they could assist with communicating the intended research message in the language that the target population was familiar with. That was a good idea, and that could assist in getting a good response rate because by involving members of the communities in conducting the research, there is a good chance of gaining the buy-in and trust of the population of interest for your research.

However, there could also be a downside in selecting certain members of the communities to assist with the research because this could potentially be viewed as a hidden agenda by some, especially if the target population is deeply divided or not homogeneous. I see such a challenge in many parts of the middle- and low-income countries where politics and/or religion and/or ethnicity and/or social class seem to stifle progress in many aspects, especially if the progress is initiated from the "other side" of the political, religious, ethnic or social class divide. Sometimes, the divide is directly or indirectly perpetrated by some of the high-income or donor countries who have their own interests in the middle- and/or low-income countries.

Perhaps, the best way to win the trust of polarised communities in the middle- and low-income countries is to begin by getting endorsement of the traditional leaders who tend to play a neutral and unifying role in such communities. Getting buy-in of the traditional leaders would not only help in getting a good response rate in the survey, but it could also help with effective and efficient implementation, ownership and sustainability based on the survey findings and recommendations. A good example is that of the involvement of traditional leaders and local councils in Uganda which made a huge difference in the fight against HIV and AIDS, and this has made Uganda a good model in this regard (Allan & Heald, 2004).

Maximum participation of the target population when we conduct survey research augers well for a good response rate and sustainable implementation of recommendations. It is important to have an approach that is tailored for that particular target population as each and every environment is unique.

References

Allan, T. & Heald, S. (2004) 'HIV/AIDS policy in Africa: what has worked in Uganda and what has failed in Botswana?' *Journal of International Development*, 16, pp. 1141-1154.

Bruce, N., Pope, D. & Stanistreet, D. (2008) 'Surveys'. In: *Quantitative research methods for health research: a practical guide to epidemiology*. Chichester: John Wiley & Sons, Ltd.

Claudio, L. & Stingone, J.A. (2008) 'Improving sampling and response rates in children's health research through participator methods', *Journal of School Health*, 78 (8), pp. 445-451.

Chopra, M., Lawn, J.E., Sanders, D., Barron, P., Abdool-Karim; Q., Flisher, A.J., Mayosi, B.M., Tollman, S.M., Churchyard, G. & Coovadia, H. (2009) 'Achieving the health millennium development goals for South Africa: challenges and priorities', *The Lancet*, 374 (9694), pp.1023-1031.

Christensen, L.B. (2007) 'Reliability and validity in experimental research'. In: *Experimental methodology*. Boston: Pearson

Cromar, N., Cameron, S. & Fallowfield, H. (2006) 'Environmental epidemiology'. In: Environmental health in Australia and New Zealand. Melbourne: Oxford University Press.

De Haan, M. (2005) 'Health needs through the lifespan'. In: *The health of Southern Africa*. Cape Town: Juta Academic.

Draugalis, J.R. & Plaza, C.M. (2009) 'Best practices for survey research reports revisited: implications of target population, probability sampling, and response rate', *American Journal of Pharmaceutical Education*, 73 (8), pp. 142-149.

Grava-Gubins, I. & Scott, S. (2008) 'Effects of various methodologic strategies: survey response rates among Canadian physicians and physicians-in-training', *Canadian Family Physician*, 54 (10), pp. 1424-1430.

Igboamalu, C. & Govender, I. (2013) 'Contraceptive knowledge and practices among pregnant females in Lower Umfolozi District War Memorial Hospital, KwaZulu-Natal', *Occupational Health Southern Africa*, 19 (1), pp. 26-31.

Johnson, A.M., Mercer, C.H., Erens, B., Copas, A.J., McManus, S., Wellings, K., Fenton, K.A., Korovessis, C., Macdowall, W., Nanchabal, K., Purdon, S. & Field, J. (2001) 'Sexual behavior in Britain: partnerships, practices, and HIV risk behaviours', *The Lancet*, 358 (9296), pp. 1835-1842.

Joubert, G. & Ehrlich, R. (2007) *Epidemiology: a research manual for South Africa*. 2nd ed. Cape Town: Oxford University Press Southern Africa.

Maree, K. (2010) 'Statistical analysis II: inferential statistics'. In: *First steps in research*. Pretoria: Van Schaik.

McCarty, C. (2003) 'Differences in response rates using most recent versus final dispositions in telephone surveys', *Public Opinion Quarterly*, 67, pp. 396-406.

Mosavel, M., Simon, C., Van Stade, D. & Buchbinder, M. (2005) 'Community-based participatory research (CBPR) in South Africa: engaging multiple constituents to shape the research question', *Social Science & Medicine*, 61 (12), pp. 2577-2587.

Mouton, J. (2002) 'Data collection (sources of error)'. In: *Understanding social research*. Pretoria: Van Schaik.

O'Rourke, D. & Blair, J. (1983) 'Improving random respondent selection in telephone surveys', *Journal of Marketing Research*, XX, pp. 428-432.

Ohenjo, N., Wills, R., Jackson, D., Nettleton, C., Good, K. & Mugarura, B. (2006) 'Health of indigenous people in Africa', *The Lancet*, 367(9526), pp. 1937-1946.

Robins, J.M., Rotnitzky, A. & Scharfstein, D.O. (2000) 'Sensitivity analysis for selection bias and unmeasured confounding in missing data and causal inference models', *The IMA Volumes in Mathematics and its Applications*, 116, pp. 1-94.

Roth, T., Coulouvrat, C., Hajak, G., Lakoma, M.D., Sampson, N., Shahly, V., Shillington, A.C., Stephenson, J.J., Walsh, J.K. & Kessler, R.C. (2011) 'Prevalence and perceived health associated with insomnia based on DSM-IV-TR; international statistical classification of diseases and related health problems, tenth revision; and research diagnostic criteria/international classification of sleep disorders, second edition criteria: results from the America insomnia survey', *Biological Psychiatry*, 69, pp. 592-600.

Scott, A., Jeon, S., Joyce, C.M., Humphreys, J.S., Kalb, G., Witt, J. & Leahy, A. (2011) 'A randomized trial and economic evaluation of the effect of response mode on response rate, response bias, and item non-response in a survey of doctors', *BMC Medical Research Methodology*, 11, p. 126.

Sturgis, P., Smith, P. & Hughes, G. (2006) *A study of suitable methods for raising response rates in school surveys* [Online]. Department for Education and Skills. United Kingdom.

Thorpe, C., Ryan, B., MacLean, S.L, Stewart, M., Brown, J.B., Reid, G.J. & Harris, S. (2008) 'How to obtain excellent response rates when surveying physicians', *Family Practice*, 26 (1), pp. 65-68.

VanGeest, J.B., Johnson, T.P. & Welch, V.L. (2007) 'Methodologies for improving response rates in surveys of physicians: a systematic review', *Evaluating Health Professionals*, 30 (4), pp. 303-321.

Welman, C., Kruger, F. & Mitchell, B. (2005) 'Population and sampling types'. In: *Research methods*. 3rd ed. Cape Town: Oxford University Press.

Whittmore, R. & Knafl, K. (2005) 'The integrative review: updated methodology', *Journal of Advanced Nursing*, 52 (5), pp. 546-553.

Woolf, S.H., Rothemich, S.F., Johnson, R.E. & Marsland, D.W. (2000) 'Selection bias from requiring patients to give consent to examine data for health services research', *Archives of Family Medicine*, 9 (10), pp. 1111-1118.

Chapter 4

Cohort Studies

The discussions covered in this chapter will cover the following topics:

- A cohort study design
- Information analysis scenario of a cohort study versus case control study

4.1 A cohort study design

LET US FOCUS ON THE strengths and weaknesses of the choice of a cohort study design in addressing the question of whether alcohol consumption is associated with the onset of dementia. A cohort study is a type of epidemiologic study and is also known as a follow-up study or a longitudinal study of disease incidence, and the follow-up may be prospective or retrospective (Cromar et al, 2006).

It is considered as the main strength of cohort studies that they have the capacity to study change and development of outcome over a time period, which gives the researcher a measure of control over the variables being studied and to assess a range of outcomes associated with the exposure being studied (Saunders et al, 2003).The fact that there is case ascertainment in cohort studies is a strength because this ensures that there is better quality data collected, which means that it is very likely known with certainty that the exposure preceded the disease, considering the possible causal relationship between exposure and disease (Bruce et al, 2008). In this regard, the fact that the relative risk of onset of dementia as a result of alcohol consumption can be directly measured during the course of a cohort study can also be considered as the strength of the choice of a cohort study design (Joubert & Ehrlich, 2007). Unlike a prospective cohort study, it is a strength that a retrospective cohort study may be quicker to conduct as it makes use of historically completed data (Joubert & Ehrlich, 2007). Retrospective cohort studies are useful if good historical records are available about the exposure and outcome, otherwise, this could be a weakness.

A prospective cohort study's major weakness is that it may be time-consuming, demanding and expensive to follow-up cases to see if they develop dementia because some of the people in the cohort may be lost due to death, relocation or refusal to continue participating before the cohort study is concluded (Christensen, 2007). The observation by Walker & Shaper (1984) that it is a challenge to obtain accurate mortality data and more so, morbidity data, is a valid point because accurate medical record keeping is a major issue in the sub-Saharan region, and this could pose a major challenge when conducting cohort studies. A very large sample could be required if alcoholic dementia is rare in the population of interest (Joubert & Ehrlich, 2007). The fact that the level of alcohol consumption could change during the course of the cohort study, and that there could be a long time between exposure and outcome could be a potential source of random error and or bias (Bruce et al, 2008). It is interesting that some authors observe that a cohort study design is not representative of the population, because different samples of the population could yield different relative risks of the association between alcohol consumption and the onset of dementia (Welman et al, 2003).

The strengths and weaknesses of the choice of a cohort study to investigate the association between alcohol consumption and dementia indicate that it may be necessary for the researchers to justify the choice of the cohort study. Confounding factors should not be ignored when investigating the association between exposure and outcome (Wannamethee et al, 2001).

The researchers need to decide whether a prospective cohort study design or a retrospective study design would be the most appropriate to use in investigating whether alcohol consumption is associated with the onset of dementia. For instance, if the researchers have budget constraints and cannot afford to study or follow-up a very large sample, a retrospective cohort study design would be the most appropriate. A retrospective cohort study is usually less expensive than a prospective cohort study design and it shortens the time needed to conduct a cohort study as it makes use of historically compiled data (Cromar et al, 2006).

It may be useful for the researchers to have some prior idea of the prevalence of dementia, as it is advisable that a cohort study should be undertaken only when there is likely to be a sizeable incidence of disease (Joubert & Ehrlich, 2013). For example, literature indicates that dementia is rare below 55 years of age, 5-10% prevalent above 65 years of age, 20% prevalent above 80 years of age, and 70% prevalent above 100 years of age (Longmore et al, 2004). In this regard, if the researchers wish to employ a prospective cohort study design to follow a cohort of young men and women aged below 55 years of age, they may have to follow them for many years before they could be certain that there is association or no association between consumption of alcohol and the onset of dementia. A retrospective cohort study design may be the most appropriate if the researchers wish to investigate whether alcohol consumption is associated with the onset of dementia in a cohort of elderly men and women, but this approach could be useful if good records are available so that an association between alcohol consumption and onset of dementia could be investigated.

However, in the event of good records not being available, a prospective cohort study design may be appropriate. Suppose in 2022 the researchers recruit a total of 500 men and women aged below 55 years of age, in the Swaziland city of Mbabane, and divide them into exposure group and non-exposure group with regard to alcohol consumption and follow them up for a period of 20 years. Suppose during this 20 year period, 10 new cases of dementia are diagnosed in the group that consumed alcohol daily and 20 new cases are diagnosed in the group that did not consume alcohol daily. According to Bruce et al (2008), the relative risk can be calculated as the incidence of disease in exposed group divided by the incidence of disease in unexposed group. In this case, the relative risk of the onset of dementia among those who consumed alcohol daily is 0.5 times the risk of the onset of dementia in those who did not consume alcohol daily. If these results are real and $p<0.05$, the researchers may conclude that consuming alcohol daily has protective effects from the onset of dementia, and the null hypothesis cannot be rejected.

According to (Cromar et al, 2006), retrospective cohort studies are particularly useful for unusual exposures or occupational exposures. Alcohol consumption is not really an unusual exposure, and a prospective cohort study design would be more appropriate in the investigation of whether alcohol consumption is associated with the onset of dementia.

Another point that is worth highlighting is the selection of subjects for the cohort study. Cromar et al (2006), mention that for common risks such as alcohol consumption, investigators may enrol a general population cohort, and for uncommon risks such as occupational exposures to hazardous chemicals, investigators use special exposure cohorts. Since alcohol consumption is classified as a common risk factor, the researchers should enrol a particular subset of the general population which may be easy to follow up.

Some researchers highlight that one of the weaknesses of prospective cohort study designs is that subjects may be lost to follow-up, which could result in bias. Loss to follow-up of participants is regarded as one of the major challenges or weaknesses of prospective cohort studies (Joubert & Ehrlich, 2007). Interestingly, through follow-up examinations in 1993-1994 and in 1997-1999, and an extensive monitoring system, nearly complete follow up of nearly 100 per cent was obtained in the Rotterdam Study (Ruitenberg et al, 2002). The Rotterdam Study commenced in 1990 and it employed a population-based prospective cohort study design to examine the relation between alcohol consumption and risk of dementia in 7983 individuals aged 55 years and older, from a suburb of Rotterdam (Ruitenberg et al 2002).

Much as researchers may wish to use a cohort study design to investigate whether alcohol consumption is associated with the onset of dementia. I still wonder if the diagnosis of dementia would not be problematic, as some authors argue that there are no proper criteria to determine for sure whether the dementia is as a result of a specific exposure or it may be due to other causes such as aging, or in fact due to an overlap of a number of factors (Reitz et al, 2007). The issue of determining whether there is a causal relationship between exposure and outcome is regarded as critical, and therefore it is important to use pointers such as the Bradford-Hill guidelines that can help researchers reach a conclusion in this regard (Bruce et al, 2008).

Cohort studies may require a large sample of people or cohort, and, a long follow up time, in order to collect enough information, which should ideally yield reliable results. According to Joubert & Ehrlich (2007), the reality is that an even larger sample may be required especially if the exposure of interest is rare, and sometimes an unnecessarily larger or smaller sample size may be estimated if such a study is still new and there is no published literature about the subject.

Since research to investigate the association of alcohol consumption is not really new, the researchers should do some background work or thoroughly search published literature on the subject to ensure that they make an informed decision about the sample size. The decision on sample size is critical, and it is strongly recommended that a statistician's advice be sought before embarking on the study (Bruce et al, 2008).

Mukamal et al (2003) are interesting when they report that it is very hard to find any previous cohort studies that have addressed the risk of confirmed dementia in a large cohort of adults with repeated measures of alcohol use. It seems as if there is an issue about confirming the diagnosis of dementia especially alcoholic dementia in cohort studies. It is also interesting to note that previous studies of alcohol consumption and dementia have reported conflicting results. In fact, some researchers report that there is no evidence of any association between alcohol consumption and the onset of dementia (Ruitenberg et al, 2002). On the other hand, some researchers report that there is an association between alcohol consumption and the onset of dementia, but what is not clear is the mechanism by which alcohol consumption could cause the onset of dementia (Hulse et al, 2005). It is possible that the conflicting results of the previous studies are due to bias.

While still on the issue of bias, I notice that some researchers observe that prospective cohort study designs are less vulnerable to bias because of the large samples, matching of subjects and adjustment of results. This is a valid point, but one wonders why there is such a growing evidence of conflicting results regarding similar cohort studies aimed at investigating whether there is an association between alcohol consumption and the onset of dementia.

Conducting a prospective cohort study to investigate whether there is an association between alcohol consumption and the onset of dementia, has its pros and cons. Of critical importance is to ensure that an informed decision is taken with regard to the sample size, and to eliminate or prevent bias.

4.2 Information analysis scenario of a cohort study versus case control study

- Null hypothesis: There is no association between taking aspirin daily and the onset of cancer
- The advantages of using a cohort study design compared to a case-control study design are:

- Case ascertainment in a cohort study design makes it known with certainty whether the exposure such as taking aspirin daily preceded the onset of disease such as cancer or not (Bruce et al, 2008). Whereas in a case-control study design, it is difficult to know whether the exposure preceded the disease or not because exposure status is determined after the onset of disease has occurred (Joubert & Ehrlich, 2007).
- The risk of developing a disease such as cancer can be directly measured in a cohort study design (Bruce et al, 2008). Whereas in a case-control study design the risk of exposure is usually restricted to the odds ratio and risk differences cannot usually be calculated. Moreover, information-recall bias may be a problem in case-control studies because the cases may not really remember all the exposures that they were exposed to especially if the exposures happened many years ago (Joubert & Ehrlich, 2007).
- A cohort study design enables the assessment of a range of diseases associated with the exposure such as taking aspirin daily being studied (Bruce et al, 2008). Whereas in a case-control study a range of exposures may be associated with the single outcome such as cancer (Joubert & Ehrlich, 2007).

The disadvantages of using a cohort study design compared to a case-control study design are:

- A prospective cohort study design may be time-consuming and expensive as it may require following-up on the selected group of elderly men and elderly women being surveyed for an extended period especially if the cancers occur a long time after the exposure (Cromar et al, 2006). Whereas, in a case-control study, there is no need to follow-up on the selected cohort because cases are selected when the disease has already occurred (Joubert & Ehrlich, 2007).
- A cohort study design may require a very large sample of elderly men and elderly women to be surveyed especially if the cancers are very rare. Whereas a case-control study design, does not require a larger sample, and may be considered as an efficient form of a cohort study (Joubert & Ehrlich, 2007).
- A cohort study may be prone to bias from loss of cases or inconsistent or poor follow-up especially if the cohort needs to be followed for an extended period (Christensen, 2007). Whereas, a case-control study is less prone to such bias because it does not require extended follow-up of cases as the disease has already occurred (Joubert & Ehrlich, 2007).

- A sampling frame is a complete list of the units of analysis in which each unit of analysis is mentioned only once. For example, a clinic patients' register (Welman et al, 2005).
- Case ascertainment involves case definition to ensure that a standard criteria is used define the specific disease of focus in the study. Case ascertainment also involves case finding to ensure with certainty that the right people are included in the study (Bruce et al, 2008).
- According to Bruce et al (2008) relative risk (RR) can be calculated as follows:

Relative risk = Incidence of disease in exposed group / Incidence of disease in non- exposed group

Relative risk = 40 / 141

Relative risk = 0.28

Therefore, the relative risk of colon cancer for those who took aspirin daily was 0.28 times that of those who did not take aspirin daily. Since the relative risk is less than 1, this implies that taking aspirin daily had protective effect from developing colon cancer.

- The relative risk of 1.00 implies that the risk of kidney cancer among the elderly men and elderly women who did not take aspirin daily was the same. The relative risk of 6.28 indicates that there was a 6.28 times risk of developing kidney cancer among men who took aspirin daily compared to those who did not. The $p < 0.05$ indicates that the risk of developing kidney cancer was significant, and therefore the null hypothesis can be rejected.

The relative risk of 1.00 implies that the risk of cancer among women and men who did not take aspirin daily was the same. The relative risk of 2.11 indicates that there was a 2.11 risk of developing kidney cancer among the elderly women who took aspirin daily compared to those who did not.

REFERENCES

Bruce, N., Pope, D. & Stanistreet, D. (2008) 'Cohort studies'. In: *Quantitative research methods for health research: a practical guide to epidemiology*. Chichester: John Wiley & Sons, Ltd

Christensen, L.B. (2007) 'Reliability and validity in experimental research'. In: *Experimental methodology*. Boston: Pearson

Cromar, N., Cameron, S. & Fallowfield, H. (2006) 'Environmental epidemiology'. In: *Environmental health in Australia and New Zealand*. Melbourne: Oxford University Press.

Hulse, G.K., Lautenschlager, N.T., Tait, R. & Almeda, O.P. (2005) 'Dementia associated with alcohol and other drug use', *International Psychogeriatrics*, 17, pp. S109-S127.

Joubert, G. & Ehrlich, R. (2007) 'Study design'. In: *Epidemiology: a research manual for South Africa*. 2nd ed. Cape Town: Oxford University Press Southern Africa.

Longmore, M., Wilkinson, M. & Rajagopalan, S. (2004) *Oxford handbook of clinical medicine*. New York: Oxford University Press.

Mukamal, K.J., Kuller, L.H., Fitzpatrick, A.L., Longstreth, W.T., Mittleman, M.A. & Siscovick, D.S. (2003) 'Prospective study of alcohol consumption and risk of dementia in older adults', *Journal of the American Medical Association*, 289 (11), pp. 1405-1413.

Reitz, C., den Heijer, T., van Duijn, C., Hofman, A. & Breteler, M.M.B. (2007) 'Relationship between smoking and risk of dementia and Alzheimer disease', *Neurology*, 69, pp. 998-1005.

Ruitenberg, A., van Swieten, J.C., Wittenman, J.C.M., Mehta, K.M., van Duijn, M., Hofman, A. & Breteler, M.M. (2002) 'Alcohol consumption and risk of dementia: the Rotterdam study', Lancet, 359, pp. 281-286.

Saunders, M, Lewis, P. & Thornhill, A. (2003) 'Deciding on the research approach and choosing a research strategy'. In: *Research methods for business students*. Harlow: Prentice Hall

Walker, M. & Shaper, A.G. (1984) 'Follow up of subjects in prospective studies based in general practice', *Journal of the Royal College of General Practitioners*, 34 (264), pp. 365-370 [Online].

Wannamethee, S.G., Shaper, A.G. & Walker, M. (2001) 'Physical activity and risk of cancer in middle-aged men', *British Journal of Cancer*, 85 (9), pp. 1311-1316.

Welman, C., Kruger, F. & Mitchell, B. (2005) 'Types of quantitative research designs'. In: *Research methodology*. Cape Town: Oxford University Press.

Chapter 5

Case-Control Studies

This chapter covers the following topics:

- Desirability and appropriateness of case-control studies
- Obtaining a suitable study population of cases and controls
- Bias and potential limitations of case-control studies
- Analysis of case-control data

5.1 Desirability and appropriateness of case-control studies

IN VITRO STUDIES HAVE shown that small amounts of aspirin may inhibit cyclogenase dependent platelet aggregation, suggesting that it may have clinically useful antithrombotic effect *in vivo* (Peto et al, 1988). Results that have been obtained *in vitro* may not necessarily be duplicated *in vivo* because there are many factors that may influence the outcome *in vivo*, such as the issue of non-adherence to treatment, among others. Suppose we would like to conduct a study to identify implications of non-adherence for a double-blinded randomized controlled trial to investigate how aspirin reduces the risk of stroke in middle-aged male doctors.

According to Joubert & Ehrlich (2007), randomized controlled trials, in which the research team randomly allocates eligible people to receive or not to receive one or more interventions that are being compared, are regarded as the most rigorous experimental designs in epidemiology. Double-blinded randomized controlled trials, are a type of randomized controlled trials in which both the subjects and the researchers or staff carrying out the treatments do not know to which trial group an individual has been assigned (Bruce et al, 2008).

Non-adherence could be minimized at the design stage of the randomized controlled trials by ensuring that a large sample of willing, motivated and informed subjects is recruited, and that a thorough baseline assessment is conducted with a clear inclusion and exclusion criteria and a clear follow-up plan (Bollinger et al, 2000). The recruitment of doctors in this study is important because doctors are very likely to understand the importance of adherence and the implications of non-adherence of such interventions, and doctors are also very likely to report accurate or reliable information with regard to illnesses that they may suffer (Peto et al, 1988). This is important because doctors who suffer from illnesses such as peptic ulcers or whose health condition(s) could be severely aggravated by participating in this study or who have very busy schedules that could negatively affect their participation in this study, could be excluded at the design stage of the study.

The implications of non-adherence to the study intervention are that the real effect of the intervention could either be overestimated or underestimated. If there is non-adherence, and those who do not adhere are excluded when the results are analysed, the results may show that either the intervention group or the control group had a marked advantage over the other, and this could lead to bias (Bruce et al, 2008). Drawing conclusions based on the exclusion of non-adherers could be misleading because the real effect of the aspirin could be overestimated.

On the other hand, if those who have not adhered are included in their original groups when the results are analysed, the non-adherers could result in an underestimation or dilution of the real effect of the intervention or aspirin in reducing the risk of stroke in middle-aged male doctors. At least, the inclusion of non-adheres during the analysis gives a realistic picture of what could happen in practice, as we know that some patients may adhere and some may not adhere with the intervention or treatment (Bruce et al, 2008). Perhaps, another double-blinded controlled trial should also look at females to see if there are any gender specific issues of adherence to the intervention.

5.2 Obtaining a suitable study population of cases and controls

ALTHOUGH STROKE IS uncommon below the age of 50, it is reported to be a prominent cause of disability especially among middle-aged males since they are considered to be at a 1.5 times higher risk of suffering a stroke than females (Edwards et al, 1996). In that sense, and based on their academic training and clinical practice experience, it would be expected that middle-aged male doctors to know better that they are at a higher risk of suffering a stroke especially if there is elevated blood pressure. Since elevated blood pressure is linked with the risk of stroke, it is interesting to note that elevated blood pressure tends to rise with age and there is corresponding rise in the prevalence of hypertension (Timmis & Nathan, 1994).

However, the risk is reduced even in middle-aged men who are healthy and who lead a healthy lifestyle. Since it is often said that prevention is better than cure, it would be expected that the middle-aged doctors to be keen on taking any prophylactic measures or treatment to ensure that they reduce the risk of suffering a stroke even if it is by any small amount. Of course the middle-aged doctors would want to know if taking such prophylactic measures or treatment outweighs any accompanying side effects. Peto et al (1988) observes that to answer such questions, direct evidence is needed from randomised controlled trials. One would therefore, expect the middle-aged male doctors to willingly take part and fully comply with this double-blinded randomized controlled trial aimed at investigating how aspirin reduces the risk of stroke in middle-aged male doctors. Various studies highlight the importance of ensuring that willing and motivated subjects are selected to participate in such research studies (Bruce et al, 2008). There is emphasis on the importance of minimizing non-adherence at the design stage.

It is interesting to note that some researchers observe that since there have not been many studies devoted to adherence, it cannot be overlooked that there is a likelihood of intentional non-adherence especially if the side effects of the intervention drug are very serious and unbearable over an extended period (Kim et al, 2007). One would assume that the middle-aged male doctors have had enough clinical experience to come up with different strategies of taking the drug in question in order to minimize its side effects. Walker et al (2006) report that adherence is increased if the intervention is preventative compared to curative, and even if there are side effects, the odds of adherence or compliance are increased as participants report multiple strategies to take medication.

The fact that the subjects in this study are middle-aged male doctors is very likely to increase the odds of adherence. According to Peto et al (1988), doctors are thought to be particularly suitable for these trials because of their particular ability to appreciate what is entailed and to judge the potential risks and benefits that may be associated with the prophylactic use of aspirin.

5.3 Bias and potential limitations of case-control studies

BLINDING IS REGARDED as one of the strengths of the ideal randomized controlled trial because it reduces the likelihood of bias (Bruce et al, 2008). In the context of a double-blinded randomized controlled trial, blinding is important because it reduces the likelihood of bias owing to differences in perceived response to treatment, sometimes called performance or reporting bias on the part of participants, and it also prevents assessment, diagnostic or detection bias on the part of healthcare providers or researchers (Joubert & Ehrlich, 2007).

The fact that both the subjects and the researchers are blinded in the double-blinded randomized controlled trial aimed at investigating how aspirin reduces the risk of stroke in middle-aged male doctors is particularly significant in this study. If the subjects (doctors) in this study are not blinded, they may already have an idea about the pharmacology of the drug and as a result they may have perceived response to the treatment, including the expected therapeutic effects as well as the expected side effects of the treatment. If the subjects perceive that the drug has serious side effects, they may not adhere or they may end up withdrawing from the study. According to Longmore et al (2004), the effects of aspirin are dose-related and potentially fatal. Those subjects taking the placebo may also not adhere because they may already have perceived that the placebo has no therapeutic effect. The issue here is that in addition to there being a reporting bias, such non-adherence could potentially result in underestimation of the effect of the intervention. On the other hand, if the subjects taking aspirin are excited about the perceived prophylactic effects of aspirin, they may very keenly adhere and report positively about the intervention (Peto et al, 1988). Such adherence and positive self-reporting by the subjects (doctors) could potentially overestimate the therapeutic effects of the drug (Bruce et al, 2008).

If the researchers or investigators are not blinded, bias may also creep in because the researchers may end up paying more attention to those subjects receiving the drug or aspirin and overlook those that are receiving the placebo or control. Those taking the placebo may end up not adhering, or they may withdraw from the study because of poor follow up especially if the study is challenging and long (Day et al, 2002). This could therefore result in assessment or detection bias on the part of the researchers. At the analysis stage, there could be a potential overestimation of the therapeutic effect of the drug or aspirin in reducing the risk of stroke (Bruce et al, 2008).

Blinding of the subjects and the researchers is significant in the double-blinded randomized controlled trial aimed at investigating how aspirin reduces the risk of stroke in middle-aged male doctors. This is particularly so, because such blinding eliminates performance or reporting bias on the part of the subjects, and also eliminates assessment or detection bias on the part of the researchers (Joubert & Ehrlich, 2007).

Physicians would be preferred as the target population when conducting research studies, such as double-blinded randomized controlled trials to investigate how aspirin reduces the risk of stroke, because physicians are very likely to report accurately about their health status compared to members of the general public. It is reported that the characteristics of those who are recruited to participate in randomized control trials differ from those who are not, albeit inconsistently, in ways that potentially affect outcome (Patterson et al, 2010).

This suggests that the results obtained from the double-blinded randomized controlled trial to investigate how aspirin reduces the risk of stroke in middle-aged doctors, cannot be generalized or not considered to be representative of all middle-aged men. There is a possibility that even if the results of the double-blinded randomized controlled trial demonstrate clear benefits for middle-aged doctors, the proportion of eligible middle-aged male patients who may qualify for treatment from the general public may be low due to the variable-risk benefit, raising concerns about application to general medical practice (Evans & Kalra, 2001).

Such a study may not only be non-representative of all middle-aged men in the general public, but it may also be non-representative of all middle-aged doctors, because settings may also differ. For example, results obtained from a double-blinded randomized controlled trial conducted among middle-aged doctors in a certain part of America may yield vastly different results from a similar study conducted in a certain part of Africa. Perhaps, that is why it would make more sense if large studies of how aspirin reduces the risk of stroke among middle-aged doctors were conducted across different parts of the world, to at least come up with some semblance of generalizability among middle-aged doctors, if at all (Peto et al, 1988). According to Wilson et al (2000), trials in any setting are rarely fully representative with respect to both patient and disease related characteristics. The unfortunate danger is that the evidence derived from randomized controlled trials is usually considered sufficient enough to base the general public's treatment protocols on. It is hardly surprising that some researchers argue if randomized controlled trials are really the only gold standard that glitters (Slade & Priebe, 2001).

Much as randomized controlled trials are regarded as the gold standard in terms of evidence based research, the challenge is that the outcomes cannot always be inferred to be representative of the general public. The results obtained from the double-blinded randomized controlled trial to investigate how aspirin reduces the risk of stroke in middle-aged doctors, cannot be regarded to be representative of all middle-aged men in the general public, due to the variable-risk benefit.

5.4 Analysis of case-control data

- Researchers may choose 2 controls per case because they
  might have found it difficult to decide which approach would

deliver the most appropriate controls (Bruce et al, 2008). By choosing 2 controls per case, the researchers might have also wanted to increase the statistical power of the case study (Bruce et al, 2008).

- The researchers could match controls for month and year of birth and maternity unit of birth because they might have wanted to overcome confounding by removing the possibility of studying the association between a confounding factor and the outcome (Bruce et al, 2008). This also avoids the implication of having to deal with unmatched analysis which is less efficient than matched analysis.

- The researchers asked about parental smoking history and birth weight because parental smoking is regarded as one of the risk factors for sudden infant death syndrome, and they also wanted to see whether the cases might have been more exposed to the risk factors than the controls

Variable	Cases (n=146)	Controls (n=275)	Odds ratio	95% confidence interval
Father smokes	11	45	1.72	0.94-3.13
Child sleeps on side (compared to supine)	75	104	1.74	1.16-2.61
Sex of child male (Compared to female)	105	108		2.56-6.12

Odds ratio = Odds of being exposed if a case / Odds of being exposed if a control

Odds ratio for being a male compared to being a female child = 105/108 = 0.97

The odds ratio is less than 1, and this indicates that there is no association between sex of child and the risk of SIDS. However, the odds ratio falls outside the 95% confidence interval (2.56-6.12), and this 95% confidence interval is very wide, which indicate that the estimate is very imprecise.

- The odds ratio is 1.72 and is greater than 1, which indicates that the risk of SIDS is greater among children who are exposed to their fathers who smoke. However, the wide confidence interval (0.94-3.13) could imply that the estimate is imprecise (Joubert & Ehrlich, 2007).

REFERENCES

Bollinger, C.T., Zellweger, J., Danielsson, T., van Biljon, X., Robidou, A., Westin, A., Perruchoud, A.P. & Sawe, U. (2000) 'Smoking reduction with oral nicotine inhalers: double blind, randomized clinical trial of efficacy and safety', *British Medical Journal*, 321, pp. 329-333.

Bruce, N., Pope, D. & Stanistreet, D. (2008) 'Intervention studies'. In: *Quantitative research methods for health research: a practical guide to epidemiology*. Chichester: John Wiley & Sons, Ltd.

Day, L., Fildes, B., Gordon, I., Fitzharris, M., Flamer, H. & Lord, S. (2002) 'Randomised factorial trial of falls prevention among older people living in their own homes', *British Medical Journal*, 325, pp. 1-6.

Edwards, C.R.W., Bouchier, I.A.D., Haslett, C. & Chilvers, E.R. (1996) *Davidson's principles and practice of medicine*. Edinburgh: Churchill Livingstone.

Evans, A. & Kalra, L. (2001) 'Are the results of randomized controlled trials on anticoagulation in patients with atrial fibrillation generalizable to clinical practice?', *Archives of Internal Medicine*, 161, pp. 1443-1447.

Joubert, G. & Ehrlich, R. (2007) 'Study design'. In: *Epidemiology: a research manual for South Africa*. 2nd ed. Cape Town: Oxford University Press Southern Africa.

Kim, E.Y., Han, H.R., Jeong, S., Kim, K.B., Park, H., Kang, E., Shin, H.S., Kim, M.T. (2007) 'Does knowledge matter?: International medication nonadherence among middle-aged Korean Americans with high blood pressure, *The Journal of Cardiovascular Nursing*, 22 (5), pp. 397-404.

Longmore, M., Wilkinson, M. & Rajagopalan, S. (2004) *Oxford handbook of clinical medicine*. New York: Oxford University Press.

Patterson, S., Kramo, K., Soteriou, T. & Crawford, M.J. (2010) 'The great divide: a qualitative investigation of factors influencing researcher access to potential randomized controlled trial participants in mental health settings', *Journal of Mental Health*, 19 (6), 532-541.

Peto, R., Gray, R., Collins, R., Wheatley, K., Hennekens, C., Jamrozik, K., Warlow, C., Hafner, B., Thompson, E., Norton, S., Gilliland, J. & Doll, R. (1988) 'Randomised trial of prophylactic daily aspirin in British male doctors', *British Medical Journal*, 296, pp. 313-316.

Slade, M. & Priebe, S. (2001) 'Are randomized controlled trials the only gold that glitters?' *The British Journal of Psychiatry*, 179, pp. 286-287.

Timmis, A.D. & Nathan, A. (1994) *Essential of cardiology*. London: Blackwell Scientific Publications

Walker, E.A., Molitch, M., Kramer, M.K., Kahn, S., Ma, Y., Edelstein, S., Smith, K., Johnson, M.K., Kidabchi, A. & Crandall, J. (2006) 'Adherence to preventive medications', *Diabetes Care*, 29, pp. 1997-2002

Wilson, S., Delaney, B.C., Roalfe, A., Roberts, L., Redman, V., Wearn, A.M. & Hobbs, F.D.R. (2000) 'Randomised controlled trials in primary care: case study', *The British Medical Journal*, 321, pp. 24-27

Chapter 6

Critical Appraisal of Research Evidence

This chapter covers the following topics:

- Finding research evidence
- Appraising research evidence
- Critical analysis

6.1 Finding research evidence

DEATH CERTIFICATE DATA can be of value for the purposes of epidemiological research, as epidemiological research helps us to practically make associations between information or data and risk factors for disease outcomes in groups or populations. Joubert & Ehrlich (2005) acknowledge that the notion of cause or risk factor could be tricky because most conditions require a number of causes or risk factors working together before the disease outcome could occur. It is of paramount importance to realize that the validity and reliability of each data element has to be taken into consideration (Bruce et al, 2008).

According to Cohen et al (2007), death certificates contain important information such as age, sex, race, occupation, residential address, date and place of death which could be used in epidemiological studies for the purpose of investigating possible factors associated with breast cancer. The approach would be to identify a country and analyse the death certificate data for a specific period such as the year 2000 to the year 2010, and then separate the information by age, sex, occupation, residential address, and place of death. One would conduct a case-control study, and the cases would be all deaths due to breast cancer and my controls would be all deaths other than cancer.

The strengths of death certificate data include its relative ready availability and relative low cost which would make it quicker to interpret the data; and its completeness would allow for interpretation and description of patterns of in-country and cross-country populations (Cohen et al, 2007). The other strength is that death certificate data can be used as a baseline, particularly in states or countries where the use of mammography is not yet well established (Geffken, 2000). Since all types of death are reported on death certificates, it implies that the interpretation of the data would have a lesser probability of being biased.

The limitations of death certificate data include the inconsistencies with which the variables are recorded in different states or countries (Geffken, 2000). Such variations would affect the interpretation of the data in the sense that one would not be able to confidently apply possible factors associated with breast cancer from one country to another country. One would also consider it as a weakness the fact that the recording of the cause of death is largely dependent on the physician, because sometimes the physician would just record it as a medical condition without being specific. The recording of the cause of death as being a medical condition has somewhat become a norm, particularly in South Africa and the Kingdom of Swaziland. This implies that using death certificate data to investigate possible factors associated with breast cancer could be a challenge. Hoel et al (1993) highlights the challenge posed by cancer mortality studies because of the issues of quality of the data.

Death certificate data presents a good opportunity to investigate possible factors associated with breast cancer. However, the strengths and limitations need serious consideration as these could have health policy implications.

6.2 Appraising research evidence

1. The published paper to be critically appraised focused on evaluating the use of a rehabilitation service to prevent falls in the community for older people who had called an ambulance after a fall but had not been taken to hospital (Logan et al, 2010).
2. Inclusion criteria for this study:
   a. A person had to be aged over 60, and
   b. Lived at home or in a care home in one of four primary care trust areas (Nottingham City, Rushcliffe, Broxtowe and Hucknall, and Gedling) in Nottinghamshire, United Kingdom, and
   c. Had contacted the East Midlands Ambulance Service through the emergency telephone system because of a fall but had not been taken to hospital.
3. Exclusion criteria:
   a. If the person was unable to give consent,
   b. If the person was deemed too ill to participate,
   c. If the person was already in a falls prevention rehabilitation programme.
4. Randomization
   a. The groups were successfully randomized through the use of a computer generated randomization scheme, and participants had equal chance of being assigned to the intervention group and the control group (Logan et al, 2010). The median (interquartile range) age (years) were almost similar between the intervention group [82 (78-86)] and the control group [83 (77-86)]. The proportion of

men in the intervention group [37 (36)] was almost
similar to the proportion of men in the control
group [35 (34)], and the proportion of women in
the intervention group [65 (64)] was also almost
similar to the proportion of women in the control
group [67 (66)].

   b. If any factors are not balanced, researchers should
       arrange a comparison between the intervention and
       control group in a way that avoids the influence of
       confounding factors (Bruce et al, 2008). Researchers
       should factor for or adjust for the influence of the
       factors that are not balanced (Peto et al, 1988).

5. Blinding

   a. Blinding means that the participants and study staff
       are prevented from knowing which treatment a
       subject is receiving in the randomized controlled
       trial (Christensen, 2007).

   b. This trial was blinded in the following ways: The
       assessors who contacted the participants and
       collected missing data on outcomes were blinded
       and the research staff that captured data were also
       blinded to the allocation groups.

6. The main outcome measure in this study was "rate of falls per
   person per year".

7. Since the outcome of rates of falls per person per year has an
   odds ratio of 0.45, with a confidence interval of 0.35 to 0.58,
   it implies that the chances of a person in the intervention
   group falling per year is 45 per cent less or 0.45 times the risk
   of a person in the control group. It also shows that there is 95
   per cent confidence that the odds ratio falls within the
   interval 0.35 to 0.58.

8. The researchers in this study carried out an intention to treat

analysis. "Intention to treat analysis" means that the subjects were analysed according to the groups in which they were initially allocated, regardless of the effect of intervention received (Joubert & Ehrlich, 2007).

9. Given the fact that the number of diaries returned between the two groups did not differ significantly (P=0.36, Mann-Whitney U test):

- We would want to know if there was a difference in return rates between the two groups because we would want to know if the difference was significant or not, and the degree to which the difference was significant or not, so that we can tell if there was any effect of the intervention or not, and the degree of the effect or no effect.

- Researchers used a hypothesis test because they wanted to quantify the degree to which chance variability might explain any observed differences between the two groups, and the Mann-Whiney U test was used in particular because the data did not meet the assumptions of parametric hypothesis tests (Bruce et al, 2008).

- The p value of 0.36 tells us that the difference between the intervention and the control was not significant since p>0.05

1. Two types of bias that could have occurred in this study are: selection bias and performance bias. Researchers in this study tried to reduce bias by concealment of the allocation process and by blinding the assessors and research staff who collected and captured the data (Logan et al, 2010).

6.3 Critical analysis

*THE EPIDEMIOLOGY OF mycobacterium tuberculosis and the use of
secondary data sources*

Summary:

Mycobacterium tuberculosis continues to be a huge public health issue
across the globe, and it is estimated that approximately 8.7 million
new cases of mycobacterium tuberculosis were recorded in the year
2011. The seriousness and magnitude of the HIV and mycobacterium
tuberculosis co-infection seems to undermine whatever efforts have
been made to deal with this challenge especially in resource-strained
developing countries such as South Africa. There is indication that all
countries need to double their efforts and ensure that they strengthen
their health systems to enable a sustainable tuberculosis care and
control. The main source of data for this report was the Global
Tuberculosis Report 2012. It has to be acknowledged that secondary
sources of data have their strengths and limitations, and the Global
Tuberculosis Report is no exception. The main strengths of secondary
data sources are that they save time and are cost-effective because the
data is already there. Secondary data obtained from an external source
is likely to be objective. The main limitations of secondary sources of
data are that the consumer of the secondary data has no control of
what has already been captured especially if there are issues about the
quality and validity of the data. Moreover, the secondary data may have
been collected by other people for different purposes which may lack
specificity and not be compatible with what one would like to use the
secondary data for.

Background and Epidemiology of mycobacterium tuberculosis:

Mycobacterium tuberculosis is a notifiable infectious disease that
typically affects the lungs but can also spread to other parts of the

body as well, and it is reported to be second to HIV as the leading cause of death from an infectious disease worldwide (World Health Organization, 2012). Although it is encouraging to see that all six regions of the World Health Organization have shown a decrease in the mortality and incidence rates of mycobacterium tuberculosis, the global burden of mycobacterium tuberculosis is very worrying as there was an estimated 8.7 million new cases of mycobacterium tuberculosis in 2011, of which 13 per cent were co-infected with HIV (World Health Organization, 2012). The risk posed by mycobacterium tuberculosis, including multi-drug resistant tuberculosis (MDR-TB) and extensively drug resistant tuberculosis (XDR-TB) is enormous, and this requires each and every country to have systems in place and to scale up their efforts in order to effectively deal with this enormous challenge, as weak health systems have been reported to be the main reason why tuberculosis care and control are being hindered (Atun et al, 2010).

Much as the heaviest burden of mycobacterium tuberculosis is carried by the developing countries, it is interesting to note that even some of the developed countries are facing a huge challenge in this regard. For example, unlike in most developed countries, rates of MDR-TB continue to rise in the United Kingdom, and this should be a wake-up call to all developed countries, and this wake-up call should remind all of us that more sustained efforts are required if we are to win the battle against *mycobacterium tuberculosis* (Zumla et al, 2013).

Mycobacterium tuberculosis ranks as one of the foremost infectious diseases in developing countries, and it is the cause of considerable morbidity and mortality especially among children (Nzimande, 1996). It is really a concern that the burden is highest in Asia and Africa, and that the African region has 24 per cent of the world's cases and the highest rates of cases and deaths per capita, and that South Africa is among the top five worst affected countries in the world (World Health

Organization). Along with HIV and AIDS which is causing havoc in the developing world, tuberculosis forms the biggest health problem in South Africa (de Haan, 2009). South Africa has recently been faced with an outbreak of multi-drug resistant tuberculosis (MRD-TB) and extensively-drug resistant tuberculosis (XDR-TB) which seem to be fuelled by the high incidence of HIV, as South Africa is considered to have the highest incidence of HIV in the world and the fifth highest incidence of mycobacterium tuberculosis and HIV co-infection in the world (World Health Organization, 2012). The dual havoc of HIV and tuberculosis undermines HIV and AIDS control efforts and tuberculosis control efforts in this resource-strapped country (Dikeledi et al, 2009). Although there has been some acknowledgement about the possible association between the high burden of mycobacterium tuberculosis and socio-economic status (Lonnroth et al, 2010), there is paucity of epidemiological research to confirm the exact pathways of this supposed relationship (Harling et al, 2008).

In South Africa, the problem of tuberculosis has severely impacted on the occupational setting especially in the mines, correctional services, rehabilitation centres, and healthcare facilities, most of which are overcrowded, and new cases continue to be diagnosed in foundry, ceramic, engineering and construction workers (Nogueira, 2009). The mining industry has been regarded as the hardest hit sector as studies have shown that miners and former miners have been exposed to silica dust which can cause silicosis (Hattingh & Acutt, 2003). It is reported that there is an increased incidence of mycobacterial disease in silicosis especially where background tuberculosis and HIV rates are high, as in South Africa (LaDou, 2007). The negative impact that mycobacterium tuberculosis is causing in the occupational setting is very profound because this results in increased absenteeism, decreased productivity, and increased medical and healthcare liability in many affected countries.

Discussion of data source:

The main secondary data source used for this paper was the Global Tuberculosis Report 2012. One has also used data from other sources such as the South African Demographic and Health Survey and related research studies as highlighted below. Each country supplies the World Health Reference Centre with information regarding cases using an online reporting system which automatically checks for any inaccuracies in the supplied data, and experts from the World Health Organization's headquarters or regional offices also follow up with each country in order to verify the information (World Health Organization, 2012). Since the Global Tuberculosis Report was produced in September 2012, there is a possibility that there might be discrepancies because it is possible that some countries might have submitted their data after this date.

Table 1: Reporting of data in the 2012 round of global TB data collection

	COUNTRIES AND TERRITORIES		MEMBER STATES	
WHO REGION OR SET OF COUNTRIES	NUMBER	NUMBER THAT REPORTED DATA	NUMBER	NUMBER THAT REPORTED DATA
African Region	46	46	46	46
Eastern Mediterranean Region	23	23	22	22
European Region	54	42	53	41
Region of the Americas	46	46	35	35
South-East Asia Region	11	11	11	11
Western Pacific Region	36	36	27	27
High-burden countries	22	22	22	22
WORLD	216	204	194	182

IT CAN BE NOTED FROM Table 1 that the European Region had the highest number of countries that did not report data, and this may have been due to the fact that these were low-incidence countries (World Health Organization, 2012).

Out of the 6.2 million mycobacterium notifications worldwide, the Africa region accounted for 24% of the cases in the year 2011 (World Health Organization, 2012). Interestingly South Africa had a notification of 993 per 100 000 population in 2011 (World Health Organization, 2012), compared to 948 per 100 000 population in the year 2007 (Dheda et al, 2010). It is also reported that South Africa had an estimated incidence of 600 per 100 000 population in 2005 (Harling et al, 2008) and an incidence of 218 per 100 000 population in 2003 (den Boon, 2007). The abovementioned trends show an obvious continued increase in the incidence of mycobacterium tuberculosis in South Africa. According to Joubert & Ehrlich (2007), Cape Town has consistently been among the cities with the highest incidence of mycobacterium tuberculosis in South Africa during the past two decades.

Figure 1: Estimated mycobacterium incidence rates for South Africa, 2003-2011

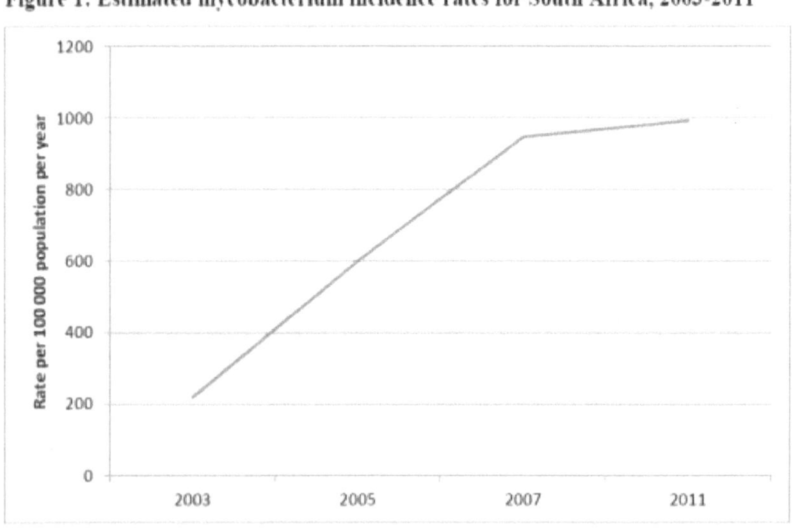

Interestingly, self-reported proportion of adults who reported having had tuberculosis in South Africa seems to be decreasing, while mycobacterium tuberculosis registration data shows that mycobacterium tuberculosis is increasing (Department of Health, Medical Research Council & ORC Macro, 2004). The self-reported decrease in prevalence of mycobacterium tuberculosis may have been due to the fact that the data in the South African Demographic Health Survey was based on a smaller sampling frame and a smaller sample size of only 10 080 households, and that the respondents may have been untrue about their mycobacterium tuberculosis history. This data was collected by researchers from the tuberculosis research department of the South African Medical Association, and the inclusion criteria was that women should be between 15 and 49 years of age and men should be between 15 and 59 years of age, and the exclusion criteria was that non- permanent residents of the targeted households did not qualify (Department of Health, Medical Research Council & ORC Macro, 2004). Such a small sample size cannot be generalized to the entire South African population. Moreover, the sample was not a true reflection of the complex demographics of South Africa.

Globally, 3.7% (2.1-5.2%) of new cases were estimated to have MDR-TB in the year 2011, and in South Africa 1.8% (1.4-2.3%) of new cases were estimated to have MDR-TB (World Health Organization, 2012). Since the p value was less than 0.001 (p<0.001) for all developing countries and was 0.1 (p=0.1) for all developed countries, it implies that the proportion of 1.8% cases of MDR-TB in South Africa was significant, and there was 95 per cent confidence that the proportion fell between 1.4 per cent and 2.3 per cent.

The number of deaths due to mycobacterium tuberculosis among individuals who are HIV positive continues to increase, and in 2011 alone, there was an estimated 430 000 deaths globally (World Health Organization, 2012). Au-Yeung et al (2011) had conducted a cross-national systematic assessment to compare the mortality rates in HIV infected individuals and HIV/TB co-infected individuals in the years 2006 to 2008, and the Pearson coefficient was 0.352, the Chi-squared value was 4.05 with a significant level p = 0.04. This implies that there was a positive linear relationship between mortality of HIV infected individuals and HIV/TB co-infected individuals. Since p<0.05, it implies that there was a significant correlation between HIV mortality and HIV/TB co-infection mortality. Since the Pearson coefficient = 0.352, it means that the coefficient of determination r^2 = 0.124, which shows that only 12 per cent of the HIV mortality is explained by HIV/TB mortality, and the remaining 88 per cent of the variation is left unexplained.

Strengths of secondary data sources:

There are a number of strengths of the secondary data sources that one has used. Firstly, the fact that the data is already there or is available saves a lot of time than when primary data is collected (Bruce et al, 2008). There is no need to spend time planning for the research design or physically conducting data collection or following-on subjects as the data is already there ready to be consumed.

Secondary data is usually less expensive compared to primary data collection (Cohen et al, 2007). By collecting data from secondary sources cuts costs of the logistics and resources needed when collecting primary data.

Secondary data can eliminate the likelihood of bias because there is no need deal with large populations or sampling frames or the determination of a sample size or complex analyses as the data is already there (Sorensen et al, 1998). In that sense secondary data can reduce the chance of bias. According to George & Landermann (1984), secondary data enables an increased ability to apply multivariate statistical techniques, and greater control and flexibility for the investigator.

Secondary data may be the only available piece of information about a specific issue such as multi-drug resistant tuberculosis. This could therefore be used as a baseline for future primary research for other settings or countries that have not had research conducted about the particular disease such as multi-drug resistant tuberculosis. It is very likely that secondary data provided by an external source such as the World Health Organization will be objective and less biased as it focuses on a global perspective.

Internal secondary data such as from the South African Department of Health and Medical Research has strength because it uses specific breakdowns preferred by the setting, and it is also easy to get more information from the people who conducted the research because they are within the country.

Limitations of secondary data sources:

The fact that the secondary data is already there, could pose problems because the secondary user of the data has no control of the quality of the data, and it may also be difficult to validate such data (Sorensen et al (1998). The fact that the accuracy of the secondary data is dependent on the person who recorded it could be a limitation because if there are mistakes, the secondary user may not be able to manipulate that data or make corrections. Moreover, the secondary data may have been collected by other people for different purposes which may lack specificity and not be compatible with what one would like to use the secondary data for.

There is a possibility that there could be missing data and this could create bias in the analysis (Cohen et al, 2007). The problem here is that it may be difficult to factor for the missing data, as we may not know the real reasons for the missing data as well as the confounding factors related to such secondary data.

It may be difficult to generalize secondary data because we may not be clear about the inclusion and exclusion criteria used (Sorensen et al (1998). Even if the inclusion and exclusion criteria were known, the problem is that such criteria may not be applicable across the board due to inconsistencies of recording such data in different settings or countries. It is possible that secondary data may only show the internal characteristics of a setting or country, and such internal characteristics may not necessarily be extrapolated to describe the entire world as a whole (Sorensen et al (1998). Such variations may occur between provinces within a country, between countries or between regions or continents.

Conclusion

The magnitude of the problem posed by mycobacterium tuberculosis is so enormous that it requires a concerted effort from all countries. Unfortunately, the present scenario indicates that not many countries have strengthened their health systems, and as a result many countries have been found wanting due to lack of effective controls against the spread of mycobacterium tuberculosis. There are strengths and limitations of secondary data sources such as the Global Tuberculosis Report. The main strengths of secondary sources of data are that they are quicker to use, they are cost effective, they are objective, they are less prone to bias, and the fact that the data is complete and available. The main limitations of secondary sources of data are that the user has no control over it which makes it difficult to ascertain its quality, validity and applicability.

References

Atun, R., Weil, D.E.C., Eang, M.T. & Mwakyusa, D. (2010) 'Health-system strengthening and tuberculosis control', *The Lancet*, 375 (9732), pp. 2169-2178.

Au-Yeung, C., Kanters, S., Ding, E., Glaziou, P., Anema, A., Cooper, C.L., Montaner, J.S.G., Hogg, R.S. & Mills, E.J. (2011) 'Tuberculosis mortality in HIV-infected individuals: a cross-sectional systematic assessment', *Clinical Epidemiology*, 3, pp. 21-29.

Bruce, N., Pope, D. & Stanistreet, D. (2008) *Quantitative research methods for health research: a practical guide to epidemiology.* Chichester: John Wiley & Sons, Ltd.

Bruce, N., Pope, D. & Stanistreet, D. (2008) 'Routine data sources and descriptive epidemiology'. In: *Quantitative research methods for health research: a practical guide to epidemiology.* Chichester: John Wiley & Sons, Ltd.

Christensen, L.B. (2007) *Experimental methodology.* Boston: Pearson International.

Cohen, J., Bilsen, J., Missinesi, G., Lofmark, R., Addington-Hall, J., Kaasa, S., Norup, M.,Van der Wal, G. & Deliens, L. (2007) 'Using death certificate data to study place of death in 9 European countries: opportunities and weaknesses', BioMed Central Public Health, 7, pp. 283-292.

De Haan, M. (2009) *The health of Southern Africa.* Cape Town: Juta Academic.

Den Boon, S., van Lill, S.W.P., Borgdorff, M.W., Enarson, D.A., Verver, S., Bateman, E.D., Irusen, E., Lombard, C.J., White, N.W., de Villiers, C. & Beyers, N. (2007) 'High prevalence of tuberculosis in previously treated patients, Cape Town, South Africa', *Emerging Infectious Diseases*, 13 (8), pp. 1189-1194.

Department of Health, Medical Research Council & ORC Macro (2004) *South African demographic and health survey, 2003*. Pretoria: Department of Health.

Dheda, K., Shean, K., Zumla, A., Badri, M., Streicher, E.M., Page-Shipp, L., Willcox, P., John, A., Reubenson, G., Govindasamy, D., Wong, M., Padanilam, X., Dziwiecki, A., van Helden, P., Aiwendu, S. Jarand, J., Menezes, C., Burns, A. & Victor, T. (2010) 'Early treatment outcomes and HIV status of patients with extensively drug-resistant tuberculosis in South Africa: a retrospective cohort study', *The Lancet*, 375 (9728), pp. 1798-1807.

Dikeledi, ., Soogreem, T., Kirsten, Z., Bello, B. & Dayal, P. (2009) 'Detection of environmental mycobacterium tuberculosis using rapid and sensitive conventional and real time polymerase chain reaction', *Occupational Health Southern Africa*, 15 (5), pp. 19-24.

Geffken, D.F. , Perry, M.J. & Callas, P.W. (2000) 'Association of occupation and breast cancer mortality in the state of Vermont, 1989-1993', *Massachusetts Journal of Medicine*, 5, pp. 75-79.

George, L.K. & Landermann, R. (1984) 'Health and subjective well-being: a replicated secondary data analysis', *International Journal of Aging & Human Development*, 19 (2), pp. 133-156.

Harling, G., Ehrlich, R. & Myer, L. (2007) 'The social epidemiology of tuberculosis in South Africa: a multilevel analysis', *Social Science & Medicine*, 66, pp. 492-505.

Hattingh, S. & Acutt, J. (2003) *Occupational health management & practice for health practitioners*. Lansdowne: Juta & Co. Ltd.

Hoel, D.G., Ron, E., Carter, R. & Mabuchi, K. (1993) 'Influence of death certificate errors on cancer mortality trends', *Journal of the National Cancer Institute*, 85 (13), pp. 1063-1068.

Joubert, G. & Ehrlich, R. (2007) *Epidemiology: a research manual for South Africa*. 2nd ed. Cape Town: Oxford University Press Southern Africa.

LaDou, J. (2007) *Current occupational & environmental medicine*. New York: McGraw Hill.

Logan, P.A., Coupland, C.A.C., Gladman, J.R.F., Sahota, O., Stoner-Hobbs, V., Robertson, K., Tomlinson, V., Ward, M., Sach, T. & Avery, A.J. (2010) 'Community falls prevention for people who call an emergency ambulance after a fall: randomized controlled trial', *British Medical Journal*, 340, pp. 1-7.

Lonnroth, K., Castro, K.G., Chakaya, J.M., Chauhan, L.S., Floyd, K., Glaziou, P. & Raviglione, M.C. (2010) 'Tuberculosis control and elimination 2010-50: cure, care and social development', *The Lancet*, 375 (9728), pp. 1814-1829.

Nogueira, C. (2009) 'Action on silica, silicosis and tuberculosis – WAHSA experience in Southern Africa', *Occupational Health Southern Africa*, 15 (special issue), pp. 27-35.

Nzimande, P. N. (1996) *Communicable diseases in the African continent*. Pinetown: Alberts Publishers.

Peto, R., Gray, R., Collins, R., Wheatley, K., Hennekens, C., Jamrozik, K., Warlow, C., Hafner, B., Thompson, E., Norton, S., Gilliland, J. & Doll, R. (1988) 'Randomised trial of prophylactic daily aspirin in British male doctors', *British Medical Journal*, 296, pp. 313-316.

Roesel, D. (2006) *Global TB incidence.* Available from: http://ethomed.org/clinical/tuberculosis/firland/latent-tb-faqs

Sorensen, H.T., Sabroe, S. & Olsen, J. (1996) 'A framework for evaluation of secondary data sources for epidemiological research', *International Journal of Epidemiology*, 25 (2), pp. 435-442.

World Health Organization (2012) *Global Tuberculosis Report 2012.* Geneva.

Zumla, A., Kim, P., Maeurer, M. & Schito, M. (2013) 'Zero deaths from tuberculosis: progress, reality, and hope', *The Lancet*, 13 (14), pp. 285-287.

Don't miss out!

Visit the website below and you can sign up to receive emails whenever Mbuso Mabuza publishes a new book. There's no charge and no obligation.

https://books2read.com/r/B-A-JPJL-ZDPAC

BOOKS 2 READ

Connecting independent readers to independent writers.

Did you love *Epidemiological Research*? Then you should read *Qualitative Methods In Public Health Research*[1] by Mbuso Mabuza!

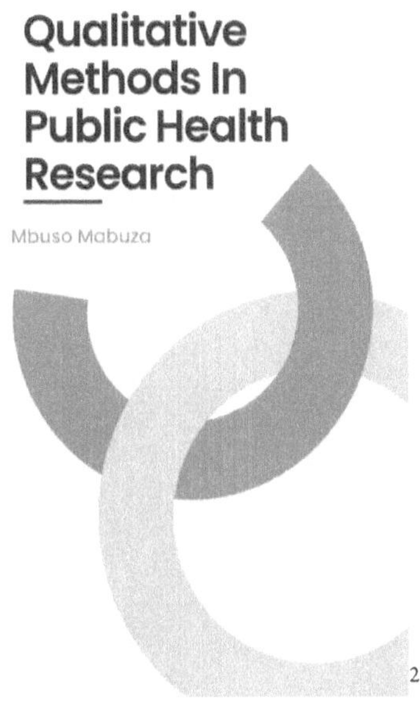

This book provides an introduction to ethics, research design as the most important part of the qualitative research process, the importance of theoretical frameworks and the relationship between the researcher and the researched in the qualitative research process.

The book is organised according to the following chapters: ethics and introduction to qualitative research; qualitative research study design; qualitative methods – participant observation; qualitative methods – interviews, texts, and qualitative diaries; participatory and action research; data analysis – coding, storing and managing qualitative data; analysis – interpretation; validity and presentation of findings to different audiences.

---

1. https://books2read.com/u/mqXzp6

2. https://books2read.com/u/mqXzp6

This book will be a valuable resource to health professionals, researchers, statisticians, data scientists, health programmers, policymakers, medical students, graduate and postgraduate students in public health and related disciplines.

Also by Mbuso Mabuza

A Healthy Mind And Best You: Achieving Great Results in Every
Aspect of Your Life
Purposeful And Better You
Sustainable Development Calls for Effective Strategic Leadership for
Efficient Health Systems
Health Promotion In Low Socioeconomic Settings
Medicine and Sociology of Health
Qualitative Methods In Public Health Research
Epidemiological Research
Ethics, Qualitative And Quantitative Methods In Public Health
Research

About the Author

Dr Mbuso Mbuza is a multi-skilled professional who has more than ten years of experience leading demanding health and business portfolios in different countries. Mbuso's expertise is in bio-chemistry, medicine, international public health, occupational health, organisational health and wellbeing, integrative and holistic healthcare, health systems strengthening and sustainability, epidemiology and disease prevention, project management, strategic leadership, research and development, innovations, monitoring and evaluation, impact assessments, editing, academic writing, creative writing, reviewing, publishing, art and design, and entrepreneurship, among others.